Presenting Toxico

CONTRIBUTING EDITORS

Graham Copping
Monique Y. Wells

Presenting Toxicology Results:

How to evaluate data and write reports

EDITED BY GERHARD J. NOHYNEK

UK   Taylor & Francis Ltd, 1 Gunpowder Square, London EC4A 3DE
USA   Taylor & Francis Inc., 1900 Frost Road, Suite 101, Bristol, PA 19007

British Library Cataloguing in Publication Data

A catalogue record for this book is available from the British Library
ISBN 07484 0476 7

Library of Congress Cataloging Publication data are available

Cover design by Amanda Barragry

Typeset in Times 10/12pt by Keyset Composition, Colchester, Essex

Printed in Great Britain by T.J. Press (Padstow) Ltd, Cornwall

This book is dedicated to my son Florian

Contents

Contents

Contributors

Robert L. Clark
Associate Director of Toxicology, Head of Reproductive Toxicology,
Rhône-Poulenc Rorer Research and Development,
500 Arcola Road, PO Box 1200, Collegeville, PA 19426-0107, USA

G. Copping
Director of Operations, Drug Safety Department, Rhône-Poulenc Rorer,
Centre de Recherche de Vitry-Alfortville, 13 Quai Jules Guesde BP 14
F-94403 Vitry sur Seine Cedex, France

S. Gosselin
Director of Toxicology, ITR Laboratories Canada Inc.,
19601 Boulevard Clark Graham, Baie d'Urfé, Montreal, Quebec, Canada

T. Hodge
Senior Pathologist, Acting Director of Pathology,
Drug Safety Department, Rhône-Poulenc Rorer,
Centre de Recherche de Vitry-Alfortville, 13 Quai Jules Guesde BP 14
F-94403 Vitry sur Seine Cedex, France

W. Kluwe
Director Drug Safety Department, Pfizer Central Research, Eastern Point Road,
Groton, CT 06340, USA

A. Lodola
Director of Toxicology, Pfizer Centre de Recherche,
Laboratoires Pfizer, BP 159 – 137401, Amboise Cedex, France

G. J. Nohynek
Principal Toxicologist, L'Oreal, Centre Charles Zviak, 90 rue du General Roguet,
F-92583 Clichy Cedex, France

Contributors

R. J. Szot
Consultant in Toxicology, 2 Rolling Lane, Flemington, NJ 08822, USA

Monique Y. Wells
Senior Pathologist, Drug Safety Department, Rhône-Poulenc Rorer, 13 Quai Jules Guesde, BP F-94403 Vitry sur Seine Cedex, France

D. Young
Scientific Writer, 66 Avenue de Generale de Gaulle, F-17690 Angoulines sur mer, France

Preface

In response to proliferating regulatory safety requirements for chemicals, pesticides, food ingredients and drugs, thousands of regulatory toxicology studies are performed and reported annually in laboratories of the industrial world. A toxicology laboratory can be regarded as a production unit, and the toxicology report as its final product. The end users are reviewers, who will use these reports to make decisions regarding the safety of the test compounds. The reviewer may be a regulator, a clinical investigator, the author of a toxicological/pharmacological expert report, or an attorney who is representing a complainant in litigation against the company based on an alleged adverse effect of the compound. No reviewer will be completely objective. The reviewer's opinion regarding the safety of a test compound will not be based solely on the results of the toxicology report; the quality of the report, its readability and presentation may also bias the reviewer's evaluation.

Therefore it is of prime importance that the results of a toxicology study, and their interpretation, are easy to follow. Consequently, writing a toxicology report is a considerable challenge for the communication skills of the author. Reporting and discussing the results of toxicology studies which may include a myriad of numerical and diagnostic results is a difficult task and requires synthesis and interpretation of multidisciplinary and complex results. However, toxicologists must keep their reports concise, accurate and focused on the conclusion which is best supported by the study data.

English has become the standard language used for reporting toxicological safety evaluations. Given the location of many laboratories in non-English-speaking countries, precise and comprehensive use of scientific English poses an additional hurdle for toxicologists who do not have English as their first language and who may have had no formal training in scientific writing.

To these ends we have compiled this Guide for the evaluation, reporting and discussion of results of toxicology studies.

We have deliberately attempted to keep the Guide simple and practical and have included numerous examples. All examples were modeled on actual toxicology reports which originated from established pharmaceutical or contract toxicology laboratories and were written by native English speakers. However, the designation, activity and therapeutic classes of the respective test compounds have been changed, given the confidential and proprietary nature of the original data. Please note that the sole criterion for selection of examples was not elegance of prose but clarity. In addition, we have compiled two sample toxicology reports, which can be found in Chapters 10 and 11 of the Guide. These examples are fictitious reports and do not describe toxicity of existing developmental compounds.

This Guide covers only a narrow range of the wide field of toxicology. Given the affiliation of all authors with the pharmaceutical industry, all examples refer to drug toxicology evaluations; examples for studies on chemicals, agrochemicals or food ingredients are not presented. However, regulatory studies performed on chemicals and food ingredients are similar to those done for pharmaceutical compounds and pose similar problems with regard to evaluation and reporting. In addition, because of the limited scope of this book, many types of toxicity evaluations, such as ecotoxicology studies, genetic toxicity studies, immunotoxicology studies and exploratory toxicology studies, were not addressed.

The principal aim of the Guide is to aid scientists wishing to improve their report writing and to propose a framework for reporting results of toxicology studies and their discussion. We emphasize that this Guide is not designed as a Standard Operating Procedure for writing of toxicology reports. It is not our intent to constrain scientists to follow a rigid procedure, or to use a standardized vocabulary or structure. Everyone familiar with toxicology studies will accept that each study is unique and may require adjustment of the report's structure, style or content to the methods and results of the study – and this may become apparent to the critical reader who may discover that the examples given in this Guide do not always religiously adhere to the recommendations of the respective chapters.

Finally, we would like to encourage all readers to send us their comments or proposals to make this Guide more comprehensive, complete and – of course – more readable.

Gerhard J. Nohynek
Alfortville, 29 March 1996

Foreword

W. KLUWE,
Pfizer Central Research, Drug Safety Department, Groton, USA

Science is organized knowledge.
Herbert Spencer, 1861

Language is the dress of thought.
Samuel Johnson, 1759

How better to introduce a book providing guidance on organizing and writing technical reports than to quote philosophers whose wisdom is ever more appreciated with the passage of time? Generation of knowledge without benefit of presentation or preservation is of little usefulness other than to its originators, and Spencer reminds us that science progresses only as the knowledge obtained is organized for universal understanding. In a similar manner, Johnson reminds us that our ideas and insight are translated to others through the language we choose to communicate them.

Communication can be considered the critical capability differentiating *live* from *inanimate*. From the most basic contact between individual cells to the complex matrices of sight, sound, smell and touch achieved by the more highly developed species, good communication describes that uncommon circumstance where the message received bears close resemblance to the message sent. Too often the message's *reception*, or its higher stage of assimilation, *perception*, differs from the message's *intent* because unrecognized failures in communication erode clarity. This invites *speculation*, a dreaded hazard in regulatory toxicology reports. More than one "battle" has been lost, or a "war" begun, due to poor communication amongst those writing toxicology reports and those assessing the significance of the information provided.

This, then, is a book about communication, and the challenges we scientists face in communicating highly technical biological information, with inferences regarding human safety, in a clear and unambiguous manner. It is a formidable task for those authors writing in their native language, with complete awareness of cultural nuances and contemporary terminology. For neither a literary education nor detailed scientific training provides much guidance on how to ensure that an audience perceives a message in a manner consistent with the intent of the presenter. How much greater a challenge, then, for those reporting in a language other than that which they normally use for daily communication? Technical reports need to state facts and provide vital information in a format that facilitates universal and singular understanding.

For better or for worse, the language most widely accepted for the exchange of scientific information, including regulatory toxicology reports, is English. Favored in many diverse countries, standard English is rife with idioms, colloquialisms, slang, jargon and terms that fade in and out of use – in short, a more dynamic language than one would have consciously chosen for scientific communication. Yet, expression of the knowledge gained from experimentation, conclusions derived therefrom, and extrapolation to the safety of clinical use of drugs is not only possible in English, but quite widely accomplished.

As described in this book, the best approach for communicating toxicology results is to first organize one's data and thoughts, then list the important points to be made, and, finally, write out the information in a format and style consistent with logic and simple understanding. Recognizing that multiple toxicology reports often follow in chronological sequence, the authors also must be wary in drawing conclusions that could be superseded by subsequent studies. Now, with the proper frame of mind, the report writer is ready to begin his task.

Readers will find general advice on how to organize the major sections of a regulatory toxicology report in Chapters 2–8 of this book. Included are formats, definitions and guidance on how to express numerical and more subjective findings in a manner that supports the authors' interpretations. The advice given is equally valuable to *readers* of regulatory toxicology reports, such as reviewing bodies, governmental representatives and even management from other parts of the authors' organization. Chapter 1 ("Basic Biomedical English") provides a concise and extremely beneficial seminar on proper use of terminology. Even those with English as a native language will benefit from a careful reading of this chapter. The very specific types of information collected in reproductive and developmental toxicology studies are addressed separately in Chapter 9, including comprehensive formats for data presentation and definitive terminology. Finally, examples of complete study reports are provided in Chapters 10 and 11, allowing this book's authors to show by example how to incorporate disparate data sets into a coherent report.

And now, let us proceed with the task at hand: regulatory toxicology report writing.

Acknowledgments

This Guide resulted from the exemplary co-operation of an independent scientific writer with a group of toxicologists and pathologists from six different toxicology laboratories in France, Canada, the USA and the UK. I thank all of them for their dedication and effort.

Special thanks to Denise Munday for her help in reviewing the manuscript and her astute and common-sense suggestions. Françoise Roquet, William Kluwe and Peter MacAnulty, who performed the final review, deserve much credit for their valuable advice and comments. I am particularly grateful to Peter for his clarification of the term 'reduction' which I (and other authors of the Guide) may have abused for many years. The contributors to the Guide, my colleagues and family also merit special mention for their tolerance and good humor while enduring my co-ordination and periods of frustration and bad temper. Many thanks to Graham Copping and Monique Wells who came to my aid when I was ready to quit. Lastly, I acknowledge the support of my son Florian (age 12) who made numerous suggestions – to his disappointment, not all of them could be included – and contributed to the progress of the manuscript by granting access, albeit limited, to his personal computer.

Basic Biomedical English

DAVID YOUNG

F-17690 Angoulines sur mer, France

1.1 Introduction

Writing toxicology reports is difficult in any language, as it involves condensing weeks to months of work into a few thousand well-chosen words.

The need to write reports in English is both an obstacle and a challenge for the scientist whose native language is not English. Yet after checking about five thousand manuscripts for syntax and overall coherence I have come to the conclusion that grammar and vocabulary are secondary problems in scientific writing. Basic English grammar is simple, and scientific prose is one of the simplest forms in any language; the general vocabulary is that of a 10-year-old child, and there is no need for idioms, metaphors, etc.

From a grammatical point of view, all that is required to write a scientific report in English is a good knowledge of tenses, comparatives and conditionals (would, will, should, etc.), a non-technical vocabulary of a few hundred words, and an awareness of words that are spelled the same way in English and one's own language but have different meanings.

All scientists who write in English read research papers in English-language journals and thus have a basic knowledge of the language. So why is it that so many scientists have trouble writing coherently and intelligibly? Clearly a large part of the problem is that scientists are rarely trained to express their ideas on paper. Often there is too little thought before putting pen to paper, and a lack – or an excess – of confidence on the part of the writer.

One pitfall when writing reports in a foreign language is the notion that vague ideas can be masked by vague word usage. Reviewers and editors are hypersensitive to imprecision and incoherence; and, as Sir Ernest Groves remarked, "What appears to be sloppy and meaningless use of words may well be a completely correct use of words to express sloppy and meaningless ideas". Data clearly speak louder than words, so once you have obtained your results, relax. There is no need to mask what you think in a cloud of conditionals, or to produce a literary work of art.

1.2 Myths

Certain myths hinder the simplification of scientific English. One is that American English and British English differ fundamentally. In fact the only valid distinction is that between good and bad style; good style is easy to understand and avoids word usage that distracts the reader's attention. Another myth is that English is better adapted than other languages to scientific writing. A similar notion prevailed some eighty years ago about German and, in the Middle Ages, about Latin. The only important difference, however, is that an English paper is about 10 per cent shorter than a paper written in French or German, for example. Otherwise a well-written paper in French or any other language may be just as clear, concise and pleasant to read as a well-written paper in English.

Today, all important journals in the field of toxicology are written in English. English has become such a standard that, for instance, a Swiss toxicology laboratory employing predominantly German- or French-speaking personnel may charge additional fees for reports written in these languages.

1.3 Brevity, Clarity and Coherence

One of the best ways to produce catastrophic sentences is to write in one's own language first and then translate into English. It is always preferable to formulate your thoughts in English before transferring them to paper. Here are some examples of incoherent thought I have come across:

- "The problem of HIV-6 pathogenicity in NHL is a few arguments in consideration of this hypothesis, which is in agreement with results of previous studies."
- "Extend experience and blood sampling should be incurred in this falling down blood flow."
- "Only hair loss is spreading with no lethal cumulative effects."

It is advisable to use one sentence for each result or idea, and the fewest possible words. However, some ideas cannot be compressed without becoming incomprehensible. This is particularly true with new methods. In this case, don't be afraid to use as many words as you feel necessary; you can always call on a colleague to crystallize your ideas.

A scientific report must be coherent throughout. The report should not contradict itself. This means verifying that sampling times, the number of animals, the incidence of clinical signs, etc. do not differ between the Materials and Methods section and the Results or Discussion. Toxicologists must not rely on the Quality Assurance Unit to correct mistakes and inconsistencies. Coherence also means keeping to the subject. This is imperative! For example, if the subject at hand is comparative ocular toxicity, then other organs should hardly be mentioned.

1.4 Internal Review

Very few scientists, even those experienced in scientific writing, can formulate their thoughts clearly and coherently on their own. All regulatory toxicology reports should be read by an independent reviewer before submission, preferably someone who was not directly involved in the study. If the reviewer is not a toxicologist or pathologist, so much the better, although a minimum scientific knowledge is required. Prior to issuing the draft report there should be an authors' meeting involving all those (toxicologist, clinical pathologist, pharmacokineticist, pathologist, statistician, etc.) who contributed to the work, and all should read the entire report. The manuscript should be taken apart sentence by sentence to remove vague, ambiguous and misleading word usage. It is amazing how many inconsistencies can be found even in reports that, at first sight, are near-perfect.

1.5 Saying What You Mean

Only state what you are certain of. If you are not sure how to interpret your findings then do not attempt to do so. If there are major discrepancies within your own findings it is better to state that "the reasons for these discrepancies are unclear". Use conditional constructions judiciously – *would, could, may, should, might* and *can* do not all mean the same thing! If you have obtained solid data with a sound experimental protocol the study should be acceptable to regulators. Above all, don't speculate – this is one of the best ways of drawing criticism.

1.6 Construction of a Scientific Report

1.6.1 Introducing the Subject

This is fairly easy. Start with a sentence or two stating the reasons for performing the study, before listing previous studies that provide the rationale for your investigation. Avoid putting your results at the end of the Introduction. Most people will find it annoying, since you already state your findings in the Summary, Results and Discussion, not to mention the tables and figures. Also, avoid mentioning the same information in the Introduction and the Discussion.

1.6.2 Describing the Materials and Methods

This is one of the easiest parts of any report. You may often adapt the text from Materials and Methods sections from previous studies; indeed, your laboratory may have standard templates for this section.

Remember that this entire section should be written in the simple past ("We did this . . .", "The drug was administered . . ."). One exception to this rule is the description of someone else's method, in which case the present tense and passive form are used: "The catheter is introduced into the jugular vein . . .". You can choose between the passive ("the drug was given . . .") and active form ("we gave the drug . . ."). Traditionalists may prefer the passive voice, but people whose first language is not English will find it easier to use the first person ("We incubated the cells . . .").

Remember that style has no place in Materials and Methods – simply state the experimental materials and conditions as clearly and as thoroughly as necessary to reproduce the work. Some references may be necessary but they should simply acknowledge the work on which your methods are based. Finally, scan the report for silly terms and pleonasms like "killed by decapitation" (use "decapitated" alone; most readers will guess that the animal died).

1.6.3   Reporting the Results

One of the main mistakes to avoid in the Results section is to repeat the description of the methods and why they were used. When the reviewer has read the Summary, Introduction and Materials and Methods and has at last arrived at the Results, he or she wants to know what happened! There may be some justification for repetition in particular cases but it is usually sufficient to state that "10 of the 20 animals died 2 days after acute dosing with PP A1101, 50 mg/kg", rather than "We administered PP A1101, 50 mg/kg, to 20 animals via the indwelling catheter after an overnight fast and found that 10 died after 2 days". If attentive readers are satisfied that the methods are sound they will accept the results at face value. In addition, increasing the reading time between the different results may lessen their flow, coherence and impact.

   All results must be reported in the simple past ("5-HIAA levels increased . . ."). This is a humble way of acknowledging that they may not be reproducible, but at least they are what you observed. Don't start sentences with phrases like "*We observed that* 10 animals died . . ."; just state what you observed, i.e. "10 animals died . . .". It is important to note that the Anglo-Saxon reader generally wants to know *what* happened before learning *how or where* it happened. For example: "10 animals died after acute dosing with PP A1101", not "After acute dosing with PP A1101, 10 animals died". (Note too that the second construction requires a comma (,), and that the use of commas should be minimized.)

1.6.4   Discussing Your Findings

There is no fixed pattern to follow when discussing your results. The only rule is that you must end with a concluding sentence or two (not a paragraph or two . . .). Remember to keep to the subject; a discussion is not a general review. In my experience a good discussion in a toxicology report may take up about half a page per page of results.

   Keep in mind that scientific research is based on simple observation. If you are sure of your findings then support and interpret them with firm arguments. You may find that your interpretation of the results evolves as you write the Discussion.

   Do not try to cover up methodological weaknesses, as they compromise the accuracy or relevance of the results and will generally be exposed in the long term. Remember too that authors of scientific reports come under suspicion when they defend their data too ardently *before* being criticized. If you have sound results, state them clearly, along with your interpretation, and let others judge for themselves.

   Avoid starting every sentence with "In addition", "Moreover", "However", "Yet", etc. If the Discussion is correctly structured each sentence should introduce the next in a natural flow of ideas. It is preferable to use words like "suggest" or "indicate" rather than "demonstrate" and "prove". Finally, do not qualify words unnecessarily, as in "unequivocal demonstration"; "absolutely clear", etc., as this is less likely to persuade the reader than to raise suspicions.

1.6.5 Abstract/Summary

Together with the overall presentation of the report, it is the abstract that will determine the reviewer's initial impression of your work. Indeed, it is often the only thing that some reviewers will read. Because of this, the abstract must be perfect!

It is generally best to compose the abstract once the main body of the report is complete, as you can usually simply import key sentences from the Materials and Methods ("We tested the effects of PP 76543 on renal histology in rats"), Results ("PP 76543 induced marked histologic lesions in a dose-dependent manner") and Discussion/Conclusion sections ("We conclude that PP 76543 damages the rat kidney"). For consistency, the conclusion in the Abstract should be summarized from the Conclusion in the main report.

1.7 Tenses

There are two forms of "simple" past tense in English: the simple past and the present perfect. It is crucial to know the different uses of these forms.

Briefly, the simple past (e.g. "showed") is used to describe actions that took place during a defined (terminated) period, such as "in 1994", "in our study" and "in the 1960s". It is also used with words like "when" and "ago" ("when we started this work . . ."; "penicillin was discovered 50 years ago").

In contrast, the present perfect (e.g. "has shown") is used for actions and states in an ongoing time frame. (Note that it is the *time frame* and not the *action* which is ongoing.) Examples are "since 1994" and "for 10 years".

What is most difficult to grasp for the person whose first language is not English is that the time frame (terminated or ongoing) is often implied. For example, all events in the study you are reporting are understood to have taken place in a defined period, i.e. between the beginning and end of the experiment (writing the report is not taken to be part of the study itself). This explains why the methods and results are written almost exclusively in the simple past ("we did", "we observed", "this rose", "that fell"). In contrast, the first sentence referring to another team's work is usually written in the present perfect ("Smith *et al.* have shown"; "It has been suggested that . . ."). Words like "previously" and "before" are generally unnecessary when using the present perfect, as it is understood that the time frame is "since the beginning of scientific research", or "since the beginning of work on this subject", neither of which is terminated.

Finally, once the present perfect has been used to introduce a subject you can switch to the simple past. For example: "Smith *et al.* have reported that . . . (ref.), but they used mice not rats. In a more recent study, Jones found that . . . (ref.)".

Note that the use of tenses must match in a given sentence:

- 'Smith *et al. have found* that LPS *activates* neutrophils'';
- 'Smith *et al. found* that LPS *activated* neutrophils''.

There follows a list of examples (singular/plural) of the tenses and modal verbs most commonly used in scientific reports:

- shows/show (simple present)
- showed/showed (simple past)
- has shown/have shown (present perfect)
- had shown/had shown (past perfect)
- will show/will show (simple future)
- would show/would show (simple conditional)
- can show/can show (= is able to)
- must show/must show (= is obliged to).

Example 1.1 A fictional, ultra-simplified report to illustrate the use of the simpler tenses in English

---

Title

PP 35824: A Mechanistic Study on the Relation Between D-fenfluramine-induced Appetite Suppression and Striatal Serotonin Levels in Rats

Abstract

We *treated* rats with PP 35824 (D-fenfluramine) and *monitored* changes in food consumption and striatal serotonin levels. We *observed* a fall in food consumption, which *correlated* with an increase in striatal serotonin levels. We *conclude* that PP 35824 suppresses appetite by increasing striatal serotonin levels.

Introduction

PP 35824 (D-fenfluramine or d-fen) *suppresses* appetite through an unknown mechanism. Jones *et al. have reported* that d-fen *increases* rat striatal serotonin (5-HT) levels (ref.), while Smith *et al. have reported* a reduction (ref). We *investigated* whether appetite suppression by PP 35824 *is* due to changes in striatal 5-HT levels.

Materials and Methods

We *treated* rats with PP 35824 and *measured* changes in food consumption. We *measured* striatal 5-HT levels by means of high-performance liquid chromatography.

---

continued

Results

The fall in food consumption during PP 35824 treatment *correlated* with an increase in striatal 5-HT levels.

Discussion

We *found* that the fall in food consumption induced by PP 35824 *correlated* with an increase in striatal 5-HT levels. This increase in 5-HT levels *confirms* a report by Jones *et al.* (ref.), who *used* identical experimental conditions. In contrast, Smith *et al.* (ref.) *reported/have reported* a fall in striatal 5-HT levels, but they *used* far higher d-fen doses.

We *conclude* that PP 35824 *suppresses* appetite by increasing striatal serotonin levels.

1.8 Spelling Mistakes and Other Typographic Errors

1.8.1 General Rules

- Decimals take a period (.): 3.47 not 3,47.
- Thousands take a comma (,) or a space: 200,000 or 200 000, not 200.000.
- Concentrations are placed *before* the compound: 1 mM EDTA, 5% FCS, 2 gl^{-1} penicillin.
- There is no space before semicolons (;) or colons (:), but there is a space after – except where a colon is used to separate two numbers in a ratio, in which case there is normally no space on either side.
- Numbers beginning sentences are generally given in letters (e.g. "Fifteen"). Some consider it more elegant to write numbers from one to nine in letters (except in the Results section).
- When writing temperatures, the space should be between the digits and units, e.g. 10 °C and not 10 °C.
- Only use metric units.
- Be consistent in your spelling; do not mix British and American spelling within the text.
- Be aware that qualitative terms are used in the singular, i.e. *increase* in body *weight*. The plural "mortalities" does not exist in English.

1.8.2 Common Spelling Mistakes and Other Simple Errors

The following exercise includes a list of common spelling mistakes and other errors. Cover the right-hand column and try to spot the error:

Incorrect	**Correct**
adress	address
accomodation	accommodation
additionnal	additional
concommittant	concomitant
conditionning	conditioning
developped	developed
occured	occurred
administrated	administered
approximatively	approximately
centrifugated	centrifuged
denaturated	denatured
determinated	determined
antibiotherapy	antibiotic therapy
comparaison	comparison
correspondance	correspondence
deshydrogenase	dehydrogenase
(the) diagnostic	(the) diagnosis
differenciation	differentiation
exemple	example
existance	existence
foetus	fetus
hormonotherapy	hormone therapy
hypertonia	hypertension
ophtalmic	ophthalmic
ophtalmology	ophthalmology
ophtalmoscospy	ophthalmoscopy
oxyde	oxide
physicochemical	chemicophysical
physiopathology	pathophysiology
(The) prognostic	(The) prognosis
radiotherapy	radiation therapy
reproductibility	reproducibility
responsable	responsible
restaure	restore
seperate	separate
signification/significature	significance
significative	significant
surrenal	adrenal
technic	technique
theoritically	theoretically
transfert	transfer
althought	although
lenght	length
naphtalene	naphthalene
strenght	strength
synthetized	synthesized
a serie	a series

evidences	evidence (invariable)
informations	information (invariable)
Material and Methods	Materials and Methods
proteins	protein
devoided of	devoid of
E. coli (genera/species)	*E. coli* / E. coli
ethical committee	ethics committee
students T test	Student's *t* test
follow up	follow-up
aknowledg(e)ments	acknowledg(e)ments
mn/min.	min
S^{35}	^{35}S
20.10^9	20×10^9
Polymerase Chain Reaction (PCR)	polymerase chain reaction (PCR)
a mAb	an mAb
biodisponibility	bioavailability
constituated, constituted of	composed (of), consisted of
encode for	code for/encode
ischemy	ischemia
Inversely,	Conversely,
produced lethality	was lethal/killed
repartition	distribution
transitory	transient
low/high quantity	small/large quantity
low/high volume/number	small/large volume/number
low/high correlation	weak/strong correlation
contribute in	contribute to
participate to	participate in

1.9 Verbosity and Incoherence

(See appendix to this chapter for explanations.)
   Again cover the right-hand column and try to find the correct or simplified form. The aim is not only to help you avoid making the same mistakes, but also to develop your language awareness.

Wordy or incorrect	**Correct**
1 pediatric patient	child
2 treated by (aspirin)	treated with
3 20 ml of water were	20 ml of water was
4 a 3 ml volume of	3 ml of
5 LPS at a concentration of 10 mg/l	LPS at 10 mg/l *or* 10 mg/l LPS
6 *X* was significantly correlated with *Y*	*X* correlated with *Y*
7 *X* was significantly higher than *Y* ($p < 0.05$)	*X* was higher than *Y* ($p < 0.05$)

8	only PMA, not zymosan . . .	only PMA . . .
9	(heart, liver, kidney)	(heart, liver and kidney)
10	(heart, liver, kidney . . .)	(heart, liver, kidney, etc.)
11	*X* was obtained from Biolab and *Y* was purchased from Prolabo	*X* was from Biolab and *Y* was from Prolabo
12	LPS could not stimulate	LPS did not stimulate
13	was found to be higher	was higher
14	LPS was found able to activate	LPS activated
15	allowed to measure PCA	allowed us to measure PCA or allowed PCA to be measured
16	was able to cause, had the capacity to cause	caused
17	without any	with no
18	we did not observe any . . .	we observed no . . .
19	treated or not with PMA	treated and untreated with PMA
20	using or not/with or not	with or without
21	in the presence or not of	in the presence or absence of
22	both by KCl and NaCl	both by KCl and by NaCl
23	both groups were similar	the two groups were similar
24	Among the 10 patients, three died	Three of the 10 patients died
25	for the analysis of	to analyze
26	protein determination was performed by	protein was determined by
27	reports demonstrating that	reports that
28	cells which had been stimulated with	cells stimulated with
29	one hypothesis could be	one hypothesis is
30	would seem to suggest	suggests
31	This case was treated . . .	This patient was treated . . .
32	healthy patients (!)	healthy controls/subjects
33	Higher compared to	high compared with/higher than
34	human volunteers (!)	volunteers
35	cell concentration	cell density
36	dose-dependent (*in vitro*)	concentration-dependent
37	10 mM of NaCl	10 mM NaCl
38	between 15 to 29	between 15 and 29
39	from 15–29	from 15 to 29
40	a 3 years old boy	a 3-year-old boy
41	the first one	the first
42	frozen at −70 °C	stored at −70 °C
43	increase of/decrease of	increase in/decrease in
44	either 5-HT, 5-HIAA or DA	5-HT, 5-HIAA or DA
45	We cannot exclude that . . .	We cannot exclude (rule out) the possibility that . . .
46	the three other	the other three
47	within the normal range	normal

1.10   Commonly Misused Words and Expressions

(See appendix to this chapter for explanations.)

Misused	Correct
1 this test needs	this test requires
2 On the opposite	In contrast/On the contrary
3 Based on . . .	On the basis of . . .
4 proteins were precipitated	protein was precipitated
5 a potential risk	a risk
6 the unique/alone patient	the only patient
7 a man having AIDS	a man with AIDS
8 Statistics (subheading)	Statistical Analysis
9 a progressive rise	a gradual rise
10 mean 27 (extremes 15–35)	mean 27 (range 15–35)
11 a raise in	a rise in
12 an important increase	a large/marked increase
13 a change was appreciated	a change was noted/observed
14 Besides,	In addition,
15 all along	throughout
16 delay	period/time (delayed = late)
17 digestive (disease)	gastrointestinal
18 dramatic	marked, sharp, striking
19 germ	microorganism
20 occasioned	caused
21 liberation	release
22 localization/localize	location (site)/locate
23 period of time	period/time
24 (animals) presented . . .	(animals) had . . .
25 proof	evidence
26 prove	show, suggest, indicate
27 punctual	sporadic, isolated
28 sensible	sensitive
29 systematic (testing)	routine (testing)
30 urinary infection	urinary tract infection
31 hepatic/renal/cutaneous (lesions)	liver/kidney/skin (lesions)
32 cellular (metabolism)	cell (metabolism)
33 urinary (output)	urine (output)
34 We didn't observe	We did not observe
35 evolution	time-course, change, course, outcome
36 e.g.	= for example (*exempli gratia*)
37 i.e.	= that is, that is to say (*id est*)
38 efficiency	efficacy
39 implicate	involve
40 In effect	Indeed (or nothing)
41 index/marker	= quantitative/qualitative
42 to control	to test, check, verify
43 this test represents a useful tool	this test is a useful tool

44 different (varying) times, concentrations	various times, concentrations
45 the surface is $10\,cm^2$	the surface area is $10\,cm^2$
46 14 days treatment	14 days' treatment
47 1 days treatment	1 day's treatment

APPENDIX: Explanations

Section 1.9: *Verbosity and Incoherence*

1 Why not "immature human creature"!

2 A patient is treated *by* a doctor *with* a drug.

3 20 ml is a volume, and is thus singular in English.

4 3 ml is a volume; there is no need to underline the fact.

5 See point 4.

6 In scientific English a correlation is assumed to be statistically significant, by definition. Also, a significant difference is assumed to be a statistically significant difference.

7 If you have stated that the threshold of significance is $p < 0.05$, "significantly" is redundant.

8 Or "PMA but not zymosan".

9 Lists separated by commas (,) take "and" before the last item (this may or may not be preceded by a comma).

10 Suspension marks are rarely used in English (and never to mean "etc".). Note the period (.) after "etc". Note too that no extra period is required when sentences end in "etc".

11 Be careful: it is important to distinguish gifts from purchases. This raises a general rule in scientific English: if you have found an appropriate word it is perfectly acceptable to repeat it.

12 "Could" is an interpretation in this phrase; what the reader wants is observations.

13 An example of unnecessary words: just state what happened.

14 You added LPS and LPS did something. Get yourself out of the picture!

15 This is difficult, even for native English speakers. Try to avoid "allow"/ "permit" completely ("We used *XX* to measure PCA").

16, 17, 18 No comment.

19, 20, 21 Avoid "or not". It is simplest to write "Animals were treated with *X*"; "untreated animals served as controls".

22 "Both by Y and by X"; or "by both Y and X". This is not important, but it is more elegant.

23 English-speaking authors often make this mistake. If you are making an indirect comparison, use "the two": "The two animals had similar lesions" but "Both animals died".

24 This is a very common mistake when describing the results. Another example

is "In the control group, 3 of the 10 animals died", which can be simplified to "Three of the 10 control animals died". Avoid starting sentences with "In" and "Among".

25   This is a general rule ("for the determination of", "for the treatment of", etc.)

26   One of the most frequent examples of verbosity. Try to start each sentence with the subject: "Cell viability was determined by . . ." (or "We determined cell viability by . . .") instead of "For the determination of cell viability, we . . .".

27   A report itself doesn't demonstrate anything.

28   Self-explanatory.

29   Don't surround postulates with conditionals. And be careful with the word hypothesis; it should mean a series of events possibly explaining a phenomenon. "LPS might damage the brain" is not a hypothesis. Try "One possible explanation is that LPS damages the brain . . ." or "We postulate that LPS damages the brain . . .".

30   A suggestion is not a statement; it is not an explosive word; don't surround it with conditionals. If your evidence is indirect, you can qualify the word "suggest" like this: "These results suggest that LPS *might* activate neutrophils".

31   Be human!

32   This is one of my favorites! But is anyone perfectly healthy, after all? Avoid "normal subjects"; they may be normal for the purposes of the study but bizarre in other respects. Prefer "healthy controls".

33   If something is "higher/increased compared to", then it is simply "higher than".

34   I've never seen an animal volunteer for an experiment.

35   "Concentration" is for solutions and "density" for suspensions.

36   A *dose* can be given to an animal or human, but not to a culture.

37   Molar is an adjective.

38, 39.   A question of coherence.

40   "A boy of 3 years" or "a boy aged 3 years", but "a 3-year-old boy". In this construction, "3-year-old" is a compound adjective of "boy".

41   "There are two possibilities: the first is that . . .".

42   It's difficult to store something at −70 °C without freezing it . . . .

43   No comment.

44   "Either" is reserved for no more than two possibilities.

45   No comment.

46   "the first three", "the best three", etc.

47   If values are within the normal range they are normal; this is why we use normal ranges . . . .

Section 1.10 Commonly Misused Words and Expressions

1 *To need* is human; things *require*. Note the difference between "require" and "necessitate" ("The patient required treatment"; "the patient's condition necessitated treatment"), although few will criticize indiscriminate usage.

2 "On the opposite" does not exist. Be careful when using "On the contrary" and "In contrast":

- "Creatinine levels did not rise. On the contrary, they fell."
- "Creatinine levels rose. In contrast, urea levels fell."

3 This is not important, but "Based on previous findings, we . . . " implies that "we" were "based on".

4 Unless you are talking about a mixture of identified proteins, use the generic term "protein".

5 In theory, a risk is always potential; only add "potential" if the existence of a risk has not been proven.

6 "Unique" means the only existing example; it is very rarely used. Use "only" instead of "uniquely".

7 Never use "having"; it's more trouble than it's worth.

8 No comment.

9 "Progressive" generally means "deteriorating" ("progressive histological changes").

10 No comment.

11 In scientific English "raise" is almost always used as a verb (synonymous with "increase"). "A rise" is synonymous with "an increase".

12 "Important" has only one meaning in English: "of considerable significance or consequence"; it never means "large".

13 Always use the simplest word.

14 "Besides" is used only in spoken English.

15 "Throughout" is a very useful word: "throughout the colon"; "throughout the study period".

16 No comment.

17 "Digestive tract" is OK, but "digestive infection" is not.

18 "Dramatic" is too dramatic.

19 "Germ" is a popular term that should not be used in scientific text. Use "fungus", "bacterium", "virus", "parasite","pathogen", "microorganism" or "organism". Note that "organism" does not mean "body".

20 "To occasion" is too formal for scientific usage. Use "cause" or "induce".

21 "Liberation" has political connotations. Nelson Mandela was liberated.

22 *To localize* is to confine. A *localized* tumor is restricted to a precise site. *To locate* is *to find*.

23 No comment.

24 A patient can *present* (to a doctor) with symptoms. After that he either *has* or *develops* new manifestations. Animals never *present*.

25, 26 Be very careful when using "prove" and "proof"; these are absolute terms: proof is unequivocal and cannot be challenged. *Evidence* is only an element of proof, and is what most scientists obtain.

27 "Punctual" means "at the right time".

28 "Sensible" is never used in scientific English (a "sensible person" is someone who makes coherent decisions).

29 "Systematic" is rarely used, and means "in *absolutely* every case". Note: "routine vaccination", "routine screening", etc.

30 See point 17.

31, 32, 33 Use the noun as an adjective when possible. The general rule in English is to use the simplest word.

34 Don't use abbreviations like this in formal text (perfectly acceptable in most correspondence).

35 Evolution generally has Darwinian connotations.

36, 37 It can be dangerous to mistake the two. Don't use "etc". in the same phrase as "e.g.:" they are mutually redundant.

38 An *efficient* motor yields a given amount of work for a relatively small energy input. An *effective* motor drives a vehicle, for example, regardless of energy input.

39 *To implicate* generally means *to accuse*. For example, "Trimethoprim has been implicated in skin reactions".

40 "The train was supposed to leave at 8 pm. In effect, it left at 9 pm." You probably mean "In fact . . .".

41 An *index* is a "quantitative marker": blood creatinine levels are an index of kidney failure. A *marker* is used to detect, not to quantify.

42 *To control* is generally *to have control of*. You probably mean to check or verify. Note that "control" can also be used in the sense of "quality control".

43 "Represent" may imply a presentation of reality or imagined reality (the painting represents a spring scene). Be simple.

44 "Different" is different from "various"; "varying" means "unstable". "Various" means "several". "Different times" means times different from those used before; it does not mean "several times".

45 A surface can be rough or smooth. If you are referring to the area (m^2, etc.) you must use area or surface area.

46, 47 Whenever the word "of" has been omitted, the possessive apostrophe is required, i.e. 14 days' treatment, or 14 days of treatment.

2

The Structure of Toxicology Reports

G. J. NOHYNEK

Rhône-Poulenc Rorer, Vitry sur Seine, France

Safety evaluation of pharmaceuticals, medical devices, food additives and chemicals is performed with a single goal in mind – to provide safe and effective products. Toxicology reports are written to supply regulatory authorities with the information required to make sound decisions regarding the risks and benefits of allowing these products to be marketed. Those employed to review these reports are not always toxicologists or pathologists. They may be unfamiliar with the type of investigation, the nature of the test compound or the types of adverse effects identified in the study. Therefore, it is of paramount importance that the results of a toxicology study and their interpretation are easy to follow. A "user-unfriendly" report is likely to irritate a reviewer, and an irritated reviewer is unlikely to develop a favorable opinion of the testing laboratory or the test compound.

A well-structured report will help the reviewer to understand and accept the authors conclusions regarding the safety of a test compound. The structure of scientific documents is discussed below.

2.1 The 'IMRAD' Structure

Almost all scientific publications and reports use the "IMRAD" structure. IMRAD is the acronym for **I**ntroduction, **M**ethods, **R**esults, **a**nd **D**iscussion/Conclusion, and is the most common labeling of the components of a scientific report. This structure was first prescribed as a standard by the American National Standards Institute in 1972 (American National Standards Institute, Inc., 1979a). A scientific report following IMRAD guidelines consists of the following components:

1 Title
2 Abstract/Synopsis: Summarizes the principal elements of the study.
3 Introduction: Why did you perform the investigation – what was the objective?

4 Materials/Methods: How did you perform the investigation?

5 Results: What did you find?

6 Discussion: What do your results mean?

7 Conclusion: What is your conclusion in terms of what you set out to investigate?

8 References

Most toxicologists would agree that all toxicology reports should contain a complete introduction, an adequate description of the methods used, a presentation of results and a discussion of their meaning and, finally, an overall conclusion. These sections form the core of a toxicology report and should thus be provided before any detailed data, i.e. summary tables and individual data tables. The organization of the report should start with concentrated information and then move on to specifics. All this is simple enough.

However, the description of the results and their discussion poses a more intricate problem. Most toxicology reports include several distinct sections, i.e. in-life observations and measurements, toxicokinetic data, clinical pathology data, and post-mortem evaluations such as necropsy, organ weights and histopathology. The results of these sections may include hundreds of findings and thousands of numerical and diagnostic results. Only a few of these data are essential for the overall interpretation of the study, whereas the great majority of them may be of no importance whatsoever. While stringent application of the classical IMRAD structure to the data accumulated in toxicology studies would necessitate a lengthy (and undesirable) discussion of *all* results, relevant and irrelevant data alike, the structure may be modified to improve its suitability for toxicology reports. In the following sections, two such modifications are proposed. Each has its advantages and disadvantages, but both may be considered to be equally appropriate for toxicology reports.

2.2 Modified IMRAD Structure

A stringent adherence to IMRAD would require discussion of *all* results in an overall Discussion section. In modified IMRAD, the Results section is followed by an overall discussion which addresses the *principal findings* of the study only. Spurious or unimportant results are addressed *within* the individual Results sections to prevent overload of the discussion. An example of a toxicology report using the modified IMRAD structure can be found in Chapter 10.

The advantages of this structure are clarity, consistency with IMRAD, and a discussion which puts all significant results into perspective and correlates the findings of different sections. In addition, this structure prevents the mixing of results and their interpretation and represents the most familiar structure for a reviewing scientist.

The disadvantage of the structure, particularly for lengthy reports, is that reviewers may already have forgotten many of the results when they arrive at the Discussion section. Thus, they may be obliged to continually flip back and forth between the Discussion and the Results. In addition, the report author who finds it difficult to distinguish between significant and unimportant results may either overload the Discussion section with spurious results or may raise the impression that significant results are being "hidden" in the Results section. Clarity of presentation of results and discussion (to be addressed in subsequent chapters) is the only way these disadvantages may be overcome.

2.3 RDRD (Results–Discussion–Results–Discussion) Structure

Using this format, the results of each section of a study are discussed *within* each respective section. Thus the description of in-life observations is followed immediately by their discussion, toxicokinetic data are presented and then discussed, etc. An example of a report using the RDRD structure can be found in Chapter 11.

The RDRD structure facilitates the interpretation of results as they come along and permits their immediate qualification according to their toxicologic significance. However, correlating results from different report sections – e.g. linking in-life findings to associated toxicokinetic data, or changes in clinical pathology to tissue changes identified in histopathology – becomes more difficult. The conclusion of the report then becomes the overall discussion section described in the modified IMRAD structure. A final phrase (or two) placed at the end of the section serves as the true conclusion of the report.

The distinction between results and their interpretation may be less clear with the RDRD structure. A simple and efficient way to eliminate this confusion is to use a distinct typeface, e.g. italic script, for the interpretive text. This method of visual distinction lends considerable help to reviewers and has recently been suggested for pharmaceutical expert reports (Matthews *et al.*, 1994).

Whatever the structure chosen for your report, a discussion among all the divisions contributing to the toxicology reports in your laboratory should determine which of these (or any other existing) formats is best suited for your needs.

3

Writing the Report Summary

G. J. NOHYNEK

Rhône-Poulenc Rorer, Vitry sur Seine, France

The summary is the most important section of a toxicology report, and as such we will treat it separately in this book. Many reviewers may read only the summary, provided it is clear and contains all important aspects of the study and its results. In addition, the summary may be used on its own or may be copied directly into databases or summary documents, technical data summaries, new drug investigators' manuals or product safety summaries. Therefore, the summary of a toxicology report *must be able to stand alone*.

The report summary should be viewed as a miniature version of the complete report. It should provide a brief summary of each of the main sections of the report – the introduction, methods, results and discussion – and should end with one or two short concluding sentences. "A well-prepared summary/abstract enables readers to identify the basic content of a document quickly and accurately, to determine its relevance to their interest, and thus to decide whether they need to read the document in its entirety" (American National Standards Institute, Inc., 1979b).

3.1 The Introduction of the Summary

The introduction sets the scene. In it, the author has to explain the objective of the study. A suitable approach is to describe the test compound and the reason the study was performed, e.g. "The study was performed to investigate the repeated dose toxicity of PP 27567, an ACAT inhibitor, in Sprague–Dawley rats". Ideally, the introduction should not exceed a single sentence. Therefore great detail should be avoided.

3.2 The Materials and Methods Section of the Summary

The materials and methods section of the summary should provide a brief review of the study design and include information on the key aspects of the study such as strain, total animal number, number of animals per group, dose levels, administration route and mode, days and sampling intervals of plasma drug evaluation samples, study and recovery period duration. In standard regulatory toxicology reports, the methods section may be limited to the description of these key parameters. It should be brief and avoid all unnecessary detail. However, any non-standard parameter evaluated or uncommon feature of the study must be described here. The materials and methods section of the summary of a standard 1-month toxicity study might appear as shown in Example 3.1.

Example 3.1   Materials and methods section of the summary of a standard 1-month toxicity study

Groups of 10 male and 10 female rats received single daily oral doses of 20, 60 or 200 mg/kg PP 27567 for 28 to 31 days. Five additional animals per sex in the control and high-dose groups were kept for a subsequent 3-week recovery period. Four satellite groups of 5 animals/sex/dose were used for plasma drug determination on days 1 and 28, at 1, 3, 5 and 24 hours after administration. Control groups received the vehicle, Labrafil™/ethanol (95/5%). The dosing volume was 20 ml/kg/day. Parameters evaluated in this study included in-life observations and measurements, interim (day 16), post-treatment and post-recovery clinical chemistry, urinalysis and hematology, and post-treatment and post-recovery organ weights, necropsy and histopathology.

3.3 The Results Section of the Summary

Only those results which are biologically/toxicologically significant should be described in the summary. If in doubt, describe the effect. In general, results should preferably be described in descending dose group order, though this is not a hard-and-fast rule. Major changes should be identified first, and the relationship to dose and no-effect dose levels should be given for each individual finding or effect. Results should always be reported with reference to the *numerical dose level*, e.g. "The following clinical signs were observed in the group receiving *50 mg/kg* PP 27567". Avoid terms such as "high-", "mid-", "intermediate-" or "low" dose. Any changes should preferably be reported in *numerical terms*, such as percentages, e.g.: "Lower body weight gain was observed in the group receiving *150 mg/kg/day*, resulting in lower body weights (*males: −15%; females: −8%*), compared with control mean values on day 28 of the study". However, please note that percentages should only be used if group size allows them not to be meaningless!

Negative results should be mentioned only if relevant, unexpected or if respective changes which are present in a high- and/or mid-dose level are absent at lower levels, e.g. "PP 27567 produced no mortality or clinical signs at 20 mg/kg/day". Any effect (including mortality) considered not to be related to the test compound and which has been discussed and rejected in the Results/Discussion section of the report should not be described in the summary.

Results may be summarized in the following order:

(A)   Single-dose (acute) and repeated-dose toxicity studies

1   Plasma drug analysis data
2   Mortality
3   Clinical observations
4   Body   weight   and   food   consumption   data,   other   in-life observations/evaluations
5   ECG, cardiovascular parameters, ophthalmology findings (if applicable)
6   Hematology, clinical chemistry, urinalysis data
7   Necropsy observations, organ weights, microscopic evaluation

Plasma drug data may be reported at the beginning or at the end of the results section. However, since the degree of systemic exposure frequently determines the incidence and severity of adverse effects, it is preferable to report plasma drug data "up front".

(B)   Reproductive toxicity studies

1   Plasma drug analysis data
2   Mortality
3   Clinical observations
4   Maternal in-life data
5   Clinical pathology measurements (if applicable)
6   Maternal necropsy observations
7   Maternal organ weights
8   Histopathological observations
9   Litter data
10   Fetal observations

3.4 The Discussion Section of the Summary

The following questions may be addressed in the discussion section of the summary of a regulatory study. They will be raised repeatedly throughout the remainder of the book as they pertain to individual sections of the toxicology report.

1   What are the principal effects observed? Is there a target organ(s) for toxicological effects of the test compound? What are the principal markers for toxicity in this study? Which dose levels are to be considered toxic; which are safe? Are the changes sex-specific?
2   Is there a correlation between multiple effects observed in the study?
3   Are the observed effects consistent with the results of earlier studies or effects described in the literature, e.g. a known "class effect" for this type of compound? Can the effects be attributed to (exaggerated) pharmacological activity of the compound? Do the observed effects resemble toxicological effects described for a different class of compounds?

4   Are there vehicle-related effects or effects related to methodology, e.g. the mode of administration or other experimental conditions? Have compound-related effects been exacerbated by vehicle effects?

5   Are there compound-related effects which are considered to be of no biological or toxicological significance? Why?

3.5 The Conclusion of the Summary

When writing this part of the summary, always keep the objective of the study in mind (see Chapter 4, Section 4.6). The conclusion should identify, whenever possible, a dose level producing no changes or effects consistent with the pharmacological activity of the compound. Key effects and target organs for toxicity should be identified. If appropriate, toxicological effects should be put into perspective (non-toxic, mild-, moderate-, severe toxicity, etc.). Generally, studies on chemicals, pesticides or food ingredients will attempt to define a "No-observable effect level (NOEL)", "No-effect level (NEL)" or "No observable adverse effect level" (NOAEL). Generally, toxicity studies on developmental drugs will avoid these terms. Given the pharmacological and exaggerated pharmacological effects commonly observed in drug safety studies, the use of the term "no-effect" level may frequently be inappropriate, particularly if pharmacological effects are evident at *all* dose levels. In reproductive toxicology (e.g. embryofetal toxicity) studies, the conclusion should attempt, if possible, to relate maternal toxicity to fetal observations and identify the dose level at which no fetal or maternal effects were observed. The presence or absence of fetotoxic effects should always be stated.

   Note: In the conclusion of studies performed to select suitable dose levels for subsequent studies, i.e. range-finding studies, maternal toxicity studies and 3-month (pre-carcinogenicity) studies, be cautious when recommending numerical dose levels for subsequent toxicology studies; new events may arise to change the perception of the data and hence the dose proposal. However, the MTD (maximal tolerated dose) should always be clearly identified.

Example 3.2 Summary of a single-dose toxicity study

This study was performed to investigate the single-dose toxicity of PP 45678, an agonist of kappa opioid-receptors. Groups of 10 Sprague–Dawley rats (5/sex/dose) received single oral doses of 50, 100 or 200 mg/kg PP 45678. Parameters evaluated included survival, clinical observations, body weight, food consumption and necropsy findings in surviving animals after a 14-day observation period.

   Mortality was 4/5 and 3/5 at 200 mg/kg and 1/5 and 0/5 at 100 mg/kg in males and females, respectively. No mortality occurred at 50 mg/kg. Death occurred within 1 hour of compound administration and was preceded by dyspnea (100 and 200 mg/kg) and convulsions (200 mg/kg only). Clinical signs (prostration, dyspnea and ataxia) appeared approximately 30 minutes following treatment, lasted approximately 2 hours and were no longer observed after 3 hours. These signs

continued

occurred with dose-related severity in all animals at 100 and 200 mg/kg. A mild, transient reduction of motor activity was noted in the groups receiving 50 mg/kg. Body weight gain and food consumption in all groups were comparable to control means. There were no treatment-related findings at necropsy.

In conclusion, a single oral dose of 200 mg/kg PP 45678 was lethal, 100 mg/kg was the approximate minimal lethal oral dose, and effects observed at 50 mg/kg were limited to mild, transient clinical signs which were considered consistent with the pharmacological activity of PP 45678.

Example 3.3   Summary of a repeated-dose (28-day) toxicology study

This study was performed to investigate the toxicity of PP 45678, an agonist of kappa opioid receptors, following repeated daily oral administration. Groups of 10 male and 10 female Sprague–Dawley rats received single daily doses of 15, 45 or 200 mg/kg PP 45678 by esophageal intubation for 28 days. Two groups of 10 male and 10 female rats were kept as controls and treated with the vehicle. For each dose level, 6 additional animals were included for determination of plasma drug levels on days 1 and 28, at 1, 3, 7 and 24 hours after administration. Blood samples were taken on days 15 and 28 for hematology and clinical chemistry analysis. The animals were sacrificed and necropsied on day 29, and principal organs were weighed and prepared for microscopic examination.

After 15, 45 and 200 mg/kg/day, PP 45678 plasma levels were directly proportional to the administered dose. No deaths occurred. Treatment-related clinical signs, considered to be consistent with the pharmacological activity of this compound, included ataxia and reduced motor activity. These were observed in both males and females; they were marked at 200 mg/kg/day and mild at 45 mg/kg/day. Administration of 200 mg/kg/day resulted in a lower food consumption (males: −5%; females: −8%), associated with lower terminal mean body weight (males: −13%; females: −16%), relative to controls. Terminal biochemical and hematologic parameters were similar in all groups. An increase in liver weights (males: +28%; females: +18%, versus controls), associated with centrilobular hypertrophy (more marked in males) was observed in all animals at 200 mg/kg/day. In conclusion, 200 mg/kg/day PP 45678 was mildly toxic, causing reduced body weight gain, reduced food consumption and adaptive changes in the liver. Administration of 45 mg/kg/day resulted in clinical signs consistent with the pharmacological activity of PP 45678, while 15 mg/kg/day had no apparent adverse effect.

Example 3.4   Summary of a reproductive toxicology study

This study was performed to investigate the potential embryofetal toxicity of PP 27567, a systemic inhibitor of ACAT. Groups of 26 mated female Sprague–Dawley

continued

rats received single daily oral doses of 0, 10, 45 or 200 mg/kg/day PP 27567 from day 6 to day 17 of gestation. Additional groups of 6 mated females per dose level were included for determination of plasma drug levels on day 13 of gestation, at 1, 3, 7 and 24 hours after compound administration. Clinical signs, body weights and food consumption were recorded regularly. On day 20 of gestation the animals were sacrificed and necropsied for examination of uterine contents, which included a detailed external, visceral and skeletal evaluation of fetuses.

A dose level of 200 mg/kg/day PP 27567 resulted in mild maternal toxicity consisting of reduced motor activity, salivation, lower food consumption associated with lower mean body weight gain (−9% lower mean body weight on day 16, when compared with control values), a smaller litter size and a lower mean fetal weight (−11%, compared with control means). In the groups receiving 45 and 10 mg/kg/day, all maternal and fetal parameters were comparable to control values. In conclusion, a dose level of 200 mg/kg produced mild fetal toxicity secondary to maternal toxicity whereas no evidence for adverse maternal or fetal effects was noted up to a dose level of 45 mg/kg/day.

General Principles of Regulatory Toxicology Report Writing

G. J. NOHYNEK

Rhône-Poulenc Rorer, Vitry sur Seine, France

and A. LODOLA

Pfizer Centre de Recherche, Amboise, France

4.1 Titles of Toxicology Reports

Imagine you are a reviewer of toxicology reports, that you are unfamiliar with different companies' jargon, and that you are not a toxicologist. How are you supposed to recognize that report titles such as "Subacute Oral Study", "Subchronic Oral Gavage Study", "Subchronic Gavage Study", "Subchronic Gavage Study by the Oral Route", "One-Month Oral Study", "Study on the Subchronic Oral Toxicity", "28-Day Study", "One-Month Repeated-dose Oral Toxicity Study", "Four-Week Study Per Os" all refer to the same type of investigation which was, incidentally, a *1-month oral toxicity study*? What would you make of a "dietary study", an "in-feed study", an "oral in-feed study", an "oral study by dietary ad-mix", or, if the study is to select dose levels for a subsequent carcinogenicity study, an "oral pre-carcinogenicity study by dietary ad-mix", or an "in-feed range-finder study"? Strangely enough, these titles again refer to the same study, which was a *3-month dietary toxicity study*.

Using a different scenario, suppose now that you have been asked to search for the report of a certain study in a computer printout containing 1500 different toxicology studies done by your company between 1986 and 1995. The study in question was carried out years ago on a developmental compound bearing your company's code number. The drug was originally a racemic mixture, was subsequently developed as a pure enantiomer, later received a common name, and was finally marketed under several different trademarks. Consequently, your computer printout contains references such as *PP 31234*, then *PP 127567*, as well as *D,L-phenyletenelol*, *L-phenyletenelol*, *Carditon®*, *Carditex®*, and *Cardol®*. In addition, the compound designation appears at the beginning, in the middle and at the end of the titles of the individual studies. Have you ever been in this infuriating situation?

The above examples are meant to illustrate that the best title for the report of a scientific investigation contains the fewest possible words that adequately describe the contents. Toxicology studies are defined by the *test compound*, the *nature or endpoint* of the investigation, the *route of administration*, the *duration* of the study, and the *test animal species*.

For general toxicology reports (single-dose, repeated-dose or carcinogenicity studies), terms should be listed, in our view, in the following order:

1   Test compound

2   Study duration

3   Administration route

4   Study type

5   Test animal species

For reproductive toxicity reports (fertility, multigeneration, embryofetal toxicity or peri-/postnatal toxicity studies), the duration of compound administration (e.g. during the organogenesis period of gestation) and endpoints (e.g. fetotoxicity) are defined in terms of reproductive parameters. Taking this into account, title terms should be listed in the following order:

1   Test compound

2   Administration route

3   Study type

4   Test animal species

For a developmental compound, use only the code of your company/laboratory, if available. This makes it easier to list studies chronologically in order of increasing compound code number. Common names should be used for non-proprietary compounds. As a rule, trademarks should be avoided. Within the title, the test compound designation is followed by a colon or a hyphen.

Avoid poorly defined terms such as "subacute", "subchronic" and "chronic". The duration of the study should be described in terms of days, weeks or months. Since repeated-dose studies with large animal numbers often have staggered dates of terminal sacrifice, it may be complicated to describe their duration in terms of a defined number of days. Therefore, the duration of studies using more than 4 weeks of treatment is best described in terms of months, whereas the duration of short studies should be described in days: 5-day, 14-day, 1-month, 3-month, 6-month, 12-month, 24-month. Be consistent when describing the study duration (note that 1 month is not identical to 28 days!). If necessary, fractions of months may be expressed in weeks, e.g. a recovery period subsequent to the treatment period (see examples at the end of this section).

We recommend the following terms to describe the route of administration:

Oral	Intramuscular	Intravenous infusion
Dietary	Intraarterial	Intranasal
Dermal	Intraperitoneal	Intravaginal
Intravenous	Subcutaneous	Inhalation
Ocular	Intradermal	Paravenous

Note that "dietary oral" is a pleonasm!

The type of study is determined by the objective of the study and its duration.

Avoid company jargon such as "pre-carcinogenicity study", "dietary ad-mix study" or "pilot study". We recommend the following terms:

Single-dose toxicity	Repeated-dose toxicity	Toxicokinetic
Range-finding toxicity	Toxicity	Carcinogenicity
Exploratory toxicity	Tolerance	Intermittent dose
Exploratory	Rising dose	Fertility (male or female)
Embryofetal toxicity	Peri-/Postnatal toxicity	Neurotoxicity

The test animal species should always be in the plural, e.g. "in Sprague–Dawley rats", "in CD®-1 mice". Avoid generic terms such as "monkey" but be specific, e.g. "in Rhesus monkeys (*Macaca mulatta*)", "in Cynomolgus monkeys (*Macaca fascicularis*)". With rodents or dogs, the strain or breed should be mentioned, e.g. "Sprague–Dawley rats", "Fischer 344 rats", "CD®-1 mice", "beagle dogs".

When the above principles are applied, study titles take the following form:

- PP 27567: 1-Month intravenous toxicity study in CD®-1 mice followed by a 2-week recovery period
- PP 27567: 3-Month dietary range-finding toxicity study in CD®-1 mice
- PP 27567: Single-dose oral toxicokinetic study in Sprague–Dawley rats
- PP 27567: 6-Month oral repeated-dose toxicity in beagle dogs
- PP 27567: 24-Month dietary carcinogenicity study in CD® rats
- PP 27567: 21-Day intravenous infusion study in Cynomolgus monkeys (*Macaca fascicularis*)
- PP 27567: 3-Cycle intravenous intermittent-dose toxicity study in Sprague–Dawley rats
- PP 27567: Oral range-finding toxicity study in pregnant Sprague–Dawley rats
- PP 27567: Oral embryofetal toxicity study in Sprague–Dawley rats
- PP 27567: Oral embryofetal toxicity study in New Zealand white rabbits
- PP 27567: Oral embryofetal and postnatal developmental toxicity study in Sprague–Dawley rats
- PP 27567: Oral fertility and early embryonic developmental toxicity study in Sprague–Dawley rats.

4.2 The Introduction

The Introduction sets the scene for the report and should cover the following points:

- A description of the test compound, e.g. its proposed use, the therapeutic class or pharmacological activity
- Location of the laboratory (for contract research organizations or companies with more than a single toxicology laboratory)

- Why the study was performed
- The rationale for dose selection
- The choice of test species.

In general the most contentious point in a study is the justification for dose selection. Generally, the dose selection should be based on the results of previous, e.g. range-finding studies, and not the results of the study under consideration. As an example, if hepatic toxicity was not found in previous studies but was the main finding in the present study you cannot say in the dose justification that hepatic toxicity was the justifying factor for the choice of doses. In our view this is self serving and unconvincing. We believe it is better to refer to principal results of previous studies or to remain non-specific: for example, "Some adverse effects were expected at ... " or "Moderate toxicity was expected ... ". This describes both the expected result and the uncertainty inherent in any study. Examples 4.1 and 4.2 are of the Introduction and justification of dose level selection.

Example 4.1   Introduction of a single-dose toxicity study

PP 24626, a metabolite of the anticancer drug PP 16569, has been identified in the plasma of rodents, dogs and man. The current study was performed to determine the acute toxicity of PP 24626 in mice following administration of a single intravenous dose. The results of the present study will be compared with the results of a previous acute toxicity study performed in mice on the parent compound, PP 16569. Mice were chosen as test animals because this species is commonly used for acute toxicity testing of anticancer drugs. The high dose level, 100 mg/kg, was limited by the solubility of the test compound in the vehicle (5% aqueous glucose solution containing 12% Tween® 80).

Example 4.2   Introduction of a carcinogenicity study

PP 83211 is an antiarhythmic agent under development for use in the prevention of ventricular fibrillation. The present study was performed to assess the chronic toxicity and carcinogenic potential of PP 83211 when administered orally as an aqueous suspension to male and female Sprague–Dawley rats for 24 months. The dose levels were selected in the light of data from a 3-month oral study in Sprague–Dawley rats using dose levels of 3, 10 and 30 mg/kg. A dose of 30 mg/kg/day produced mortality (3/20 males), a lower mean body weight (−12% to −18%) and food consumption associated with moderate clinical signs (ptosis, peripheral vasodilatation), increased urinary output, reduced plasma potassium levels, a marked increase in liver weight, and centrilobular hypertrophy. At 10 mg/kg/day, findings were limited to a lower mean body weight (−6% to −9%), a mild increase in liver weight and minimal to mild centrilobular hypertrophy.

On the basis of these results, 10 mg/kg/day was selected as the highest dose level for the present study; 3 and 1 mg/kg/day are multiples of the probable therapeutic dose and were selected to establish a dose-relationship of potential adverse effects.

4.3 The Materials and Methods Section

This section should follow the introduction. The author may choose between a detailed presentation of the methods or an abbreviated one (if abbreviated, the text should be sufficiently detailed to allow the reader to understand how the study was conducted). When using abbreviated materials and methods, the study protocol should be supplied in an appendix to the report.

A common misconception is that the Materials and Methods section and the study protocol are one and the same thing. The protocol is a "route-map" written to ensure that the study is performed according to Good Laboratory Practice and Standard Operating Procedures, whereas the Materials and Methods section is written to ensure that *the reviewer understands the study design*. Therefore, this section *should not* be a copy of the study protocol.

Whereas the Materials and Methods section can be abbreviated, all unusual study methods should be described if the information is considered useful for comprehension of the study objective or the study design. Any *non-standard* parameters or features evaluated must always be described in this section. Such information may include details of the vehicle, the administration volume and rate (key information for intravenous studies), the number of satellite animals/groups included for plasma drug analysis or recovery, particular aspects of the statistical evaluation, specific in-life observations, ophthalmology, or cardiovascular parameters, special clinical pathology measurements, details of euthanasia and necropsy procedures, organ weight evaluation, histopathology or plasma drug analysis.

Since most regulatory toxicology studies follow international regulatory guidelines which specify most of the details of the study, this part of the report can be prepared as a template which can be applied to each study of the same type. Examples for Materials and Methods sections are given below.

In some studies, e.g. those in which the test compound is given in the diet or in the drinking water, the calculated (nominal) dose levels are not identical to the actual doses administered. For such studies, the actual and nominal doses should be reviewed in the Materials and Methods section or at the beginning of the Results section (see Example 4.4).

We recommend that the Materials and Methods section of any regulatory toxicology study should not exceed one full page – even for studies having a complicated design. As a rule, half a page should be sufficient for a standard regulatory toxicology report.

Example 4.3 Materials and Methods section of a peri-/postnatal toxicity study in rats

PP 27567 was administered by oral gavage as an aqueous suspension containing 0.5% methylcellulose and 0.1% polysorbate 80 to groups of 20 inseminated Sprague–Dawley rats, from day 15 post-insemination (p.i.) until parturition and throughout the entire lactation period at daily dose levels of 15, 30 and 60 mg/kg. A control group of 20 inseminated rats received the vehicle over the same administration period.

continued

The animals were weighed and examined daily for clinical signs. Food consumption was determined daily. The number and body weight of pups were recorded and their physical and functional development and behavior were evaluated on standardized litters. On day 21 post-partum, maternal animals were sacrificed and necropsied. Developmental parameters evaluated in the pups of the F_1 generation included pinna detachment (from day 4 post-partum), incisor eruption (from day 11), eye opening (from day 15), testes descent (day 25) and vaginal opening (day 37). Functional parameters evaluated included the surface righting reflex (from day 4), negative geotaxis (from day 4), swimming development (day 10), forelimb support (from day 11), auditory startle reflex (from day 12), pupillary reflex (day 19) and rotarod performance (day 25). Behavioral parameters evaluated included homing behavior on a level surface (day 21), and learning/memory via the water maze test (days 42 and 49) and exploratory behavior using the open field test (day 48). On day 51 post-partum, all pups of the F_1 generation were sacrificed and necropsied. The study protocol containing detailed materials and methods is found in Appendix 1 of this report.

Example 4.4 Nominal versus actual dose levels

Dietary concentrations of PP 27567 were adjusted on a weekly basis; appropriate concentrations were calculated prospectively on the basis of the group mean food consumption expected to result in a nominal daily intake of 100, 200 and 400 mg/kg/day. Actual daily intake data calculated on the basis of the weekly food consumption are shown in Table 6, Appendix VI. Throughout the study, the mean actual daily intake of PP 27567 is summarized in Table 4.1.

Table 4.1 PP 27567: 3-Month dietary toxicity study in rats – nominal and actual dose levels.

	Males			Females		
Nominal dose (mg/kg/day)	100	200	400	100	200	400
Actual dose (mg/kg/day)	107 ± 23	195 ± 45	373 ± 54	110 ± 13	187 ± 32	354 ± 48

The actual intake of PP 27567 was within approximately ±10% of the calculated intake. A variation of this magnitude is considered acceptable for studies in which the compound is dosed in-diet.

Example 4.5   Materials and Methods section of a carcinogenicity study

> Groups of 60 male and 60 female Sprague–Dawley (Charles River) rats were treated daily by gavage with 1, 5 or 25 mg/kg PP 27567 for 24 months. At the start of the study, the animals were approximately 6 weeks old and weighed 185 to 205 grams (males) and 155 to 173 grams (females). The compound was suspended in an aqueous solution of methylcellulose (1%) and administered at a constant volume of 5 ml/kg. Two control groups of 60 rats/sex, received 5 ml/kg of the vehicle alone for the same treatment period. Satellite groups of 5 animals/sex/dose level were included to determine plasma drug levels.
>
> All animals were observed daily for clinical signs. Their body weight was recorded weekly. Food consumption was measured weekly during the first 3 months of the study, then every 2 weeks for the remainder of the study. Water consumption was measured over 24 hours every 2 months. An ophthalmologic examination was performed before the start of the study and at 6, 12 and 18 months. Plasma drug levels were determined from blood samples collected 4 hours after compound administration after 6, 12 and 18 months. After 24 months of treatment, animals were sacrificed, necropsied, and organ weights determined. Hematology and clinical chemistry evaluations were performed on blood samples collected at sacrifice. A histopathologic evaluation was performed on a range of tissues.
>
> The two control groups were combined for statistical treatment of findings whenever there was no significant difference between them. Groups were compared using a one-way analysis of variance. For some parameters, when a large heterogeneity of variances was associated with a large variation of animal number per group, a non-parametric analysis of variance was performed. Survival data were analyzed using the log-rank test. Peto's analysis was used to compare the tumor incidence in treated groups with that in control groups. The study protocol containing detailed materials and methods can be found in Appendix 1 of this report.

4.4 Describing Results

In our view a well-balanced toxicology report must describe the data in terms of toxicological significance; this after all is the objective of the exercise. The description of results should be as succinct as possible to avoid boring the reader. Therefore, the use of short sentences is strongly advised. Condensing complex data into a few (complex) phrases is to be avoided, particularly if English is not your first language. Remember that the first consideration in any report is clarity, and that incomprehensibility is the hallmark of a bad report.

For studies carried out with a single specific objective, such as toxicokinetic studies, or investigative studies on a specific target organ, the Results section should focus on those results which address the objective of the study. Thus the results of a toxicokinetic study should primarily focus on plasma drug data; other results, such as in-life effects, are of secondary interest in such a study, provided there are no changes which may affect plasma drug levels (body weight, food consumption changes, emesis, diarrhea, etc.).

In the Results section of a standard general toxicity or reproductive toxicity study, the author should (a) describe all effects that are induced by the test compound and (b) distinguish compound-related effects from those which are of uncertain relationship to the compound, those which are related to the vehicle or the test procedure, and those which are incidental. Given that "*treatment*-related" effects may include changes caused by the procedure or the vehicle, refer to all effects caused by a test article as "*compound*-related" effects!

Each subsection (clinical signs, cardiovascular parameters, clinical pathology, etc.) should begin with a few sentences which clearly identify the key findings. This focuses the attention of the reader *and* the author on the key points which will be raised in the discussion. Describe data in terms of incidence, time of onset, duration and/or severity. Subdivide findings by sex, dose level, or duration of treatment to help reduce the complexity of your text.

The results for males should precede those for females. Although this is not politically correct, it is general practice and expected by reviewers. Results may be described in descending or ascending dose order. The preferred option is that which most clearly identifies compound-related changes and the no-effect dose level. Within a given section the same convention should be followed throughout. Identification of treated groups by their numerical dose level is unambiguous and a reminder to the reader of the actual dose level. However, the occasional use of "high-, mid- and low-dose", while less informative, lightens the text. If an individual animal is discussed, always indicate the animal number and dose ("Male 11 (20 mg/kg/day)" or "one 20 mg/kg/day male animal (M11)"). Also, when referring to animals other than those of the main study groups, the dose and group descriptor should be given (satellite groups, sentinel groups or recovery groups).

For quantitative data always report *numerical* changes, e.g., "Treatment with 150 mg/kg/day PP 27567 for 4 weeks produced a lower mean body weight gain in males and females (Males: -15%; Females: -8%, relative to controls)" or "A *12% lower* mean body weight gain was observed". However, be cautious when using percentages to quantify changes, particularly when changes greater than 100% are reported (see also Chapter 7). There may be different interpretations of what a descriptor such as "a 125% increase in liver weight" means. An unambiguous manner in which to address quantitative differences from controls is to express increases or decreases in a parameter as a direct multiple of the control value. For example, "absolute liver weight at 24 mg/kg/day was 1.85 × those of the controls, WBC count in the 25 mg/kg/day females was 0.45 × that of the controls, body weights in the mid- and high-dose groups were 0.95 × and 0.85 × that of the controls, respectively."

A qualitative description of data in the Results section (for example, "a *slightly lower* mean body weight gain") is inappropriate since it does not allow the reader to form a judgment as to the amplitude of the change. What represents a "small increase" to you may be a "large increase" to someone else! However, the use of qualitative descriptors is appropriate in summaries or abstracts when the intention is to provide an overview of findings rather than details.

Be aware of the meaning of the term "reduction" – it implies a decrease from a known initial value. Parameters such as weight gain, organ or fetal weights can only be "reduced" if they are known to have been higher at some earlier stage. Strictly speaking, body weights can be reduced when compared with pretest values, but not when compared with control values. Similarly a "reduction in testes weight" implies that the testes were heavier at a previous time point. However, whereas terms such as "a reduction (decrease) in mean body weight when compared with control means" may not be accurate, they are commonly used in toxicology reports and are acceptable.

Findings should be graded when they are difficult to quantify or when grading may improve the reader's comprehension of complex changes. The grading scheme should be defined in the text or as a footnote to the data. A three-grade (mild – moderate – severe) or five-grade system (minimal – mild – moderate – marked – severe) is generally used (see Table 4.2 below).

The statistical significance of change should be described in the text, e.g. "A statistically significant decrease in mean WBC count occurred in males treated with 100 mg/kg/day". Alternatively, p-values may be used to indicate statistical significance. For example: "There was a decrease ($p < 0.01$) in mean WBC count in males treated with 100 mg/kg/day". While there is no set rule, inclusion of p-values lightens the text and facilitates reading.

Often, the simplest way of describing complex results is by using a table. Tables should be numbered and preceded by a title. The title relates the purpose and the contents of the table. The title, the footnotes and the column headings together should form a complete unit that is independent of the text. Any abbreviation must be explained in a footnote. The order of data presentation should always be from control to high dose. An example is given in Example 4.6.

Example 4.6   Tabular presentation of results

Table 4.2   PP 27567: 1-Month oral toxicity in dogs – incidence and severity of intra-canalicular cholestasis.

Severity of cholestasis	Controls		10 mg/kg		40 mg/kg		120 mg/kg	
	males	females	males	females	males	females	males	females
mild	0/4	0/4	1/4	1/4	1/4	2/4	0/4	0/4
moderate	0/4	0/4	0/4	1/4	0/4	1/4	1/4	1/4
severe	0/4	0/4	0/4	0/4	1/4	1/4	3/4	2/4

Grading system: *mild*: focal centrilobular change, comprising up to 5 bile plugs per liver section; *moderate*: multifocal centrilobular change, comprising more than 5 but less than 20 bile plugs per liver section; *severe*: >20 bile plugs, presenting as a zonal change affecting most centrilobular areas.

In-life observations or other data from satellite groups (e.g. for plasma drug determination) should not be described within the Results section, unless specified in the protocol. Exceptions are pregnancy data in fertility study satellite groups and compound-related mortality data. Note that mortality in rodent satellite groups which may be attributed to anesthesia and/or blood sampling procedure and which occur in absence of mortality in the main groups should be described as *procedure-related* mortality, but not as *compound-related* mortality! Again, avoid the potentially confusing term "treatment-related" mortality!

The absence of an effect on an individual parameter which was measured in the study should always be mentioned, e.g.: "There was no effect on body weight or food consumption", or "No changes were detected in blood pressure or heart rates". If changes are evident at the high- and/or mid-dose level, but not at a lower dose level, the absence of an effect should be mentioned with reference to the dose level where the effect was absent. Always conclude any description of compound-related effects with an appropriate phrase highlighting the no-effect dose level, e.g. "A reduction in mean body weight was noted in the male group receiving 150 mg/kg (−9%, when compared with the control mean). The body weights of all other treated groups were comparable to control values." The same rule applies if effects that were anticipated were not observed, e.g. on the basis of the results of previous studies or on the pharmacological activity of the test compound.

The reasons for dismissing findings which might be considered to be compound-related should be given in the Results section (this is our personal preference, as it simplifies the discussion and focuses it on the issues) or in the Discussion. In general, data are dismissed on the basis of the *absence of a dose response, isolated occurrence, and/or being within the limits of historical control data*. A brief statement such as "All other findings were those which routinely occur in our laboratory in rats/dogs of this age, sex and strain" is also useful in assuring the reader that all the data have been reviewed to identify treatment-related changes.

4.5 The Evaluation/Discussion Section

The extent to which the results of a regulatory toxicity study should be discussed is a controversial topic. Some laboratories do not include a discussion in reports, or keep the discussion of the results to a minimum. Their appraisal of toxic effects is done in the Toxicological Expert Review or Synopsis where the results from all studies are discussed; this approach avoids discussion of spurious effects in early studies and speculation as to the pathogenesis of confirmed toxic effects.

Alternatively, the principal results of individual toxicity studies can be discussed extensively in each report. Individual study reports are frequently reviewed independently of the toxicological expert report, and discussion within each report allays the concern that the findings of a given study may be misinterpreted by a naive reviewer. While the extent of the discussion is debatable, in our view it is preferable to discuss the results of each study within the report itself.

The principal themes that should be addressed in the discussion include the following.

- **Study objective**: Focus the discussion on the study objective. You don't need a detailed discussion of in-life effects in a toxicokinetic study (provided such effects did not affect the plasma drug levels)!

- **Principal effects**: What are the principal effects observed in this study? Are there principal target organs for the test compound? What are the principal markers for toxicity in this study? Which doses are toxic? Are effects sex-specific?

- **Correlation of effects**: Is there a correlation between effects observed in the study?

- **Pathogenesis**: Are the effects consistent with the results of earlier studies or effects described in the literature? Is the pathogenesis of the effects known? Is it a "class effect"? Are the effects caused by the exaggerated pharmacological activity of the compound? Are the effects relevant to man?

Vehicle-related effects and effects related to the method of compound administration should be discussed after these points have been addressed. Compound-related effects which are considered to be biologically or toxicologically insignificant (provided they have not been dismissed in the Results section) should also be discussed at this time.

There are no hard-and-fast rules governing the ordering of facts in the Discussion. Findings can be discussed in increasing or decreasing order of importance, or in the same order in which they occur in the Results. Whichever approach is preferred, discuss your results, do not repeat them! Keep your language and your ideas as simple as possible; remember to KISS (**K**eep **I**t **S**hort and **S**imple!) the text. Also, remember that, as the pre-clinical safety program unfolds, what appeared to be of major significance in early studies can be of little or no relevance in later studies. Therefore, avoid speculation unless it is based on a solid scientific foundation. It is preferable to leave a point open rather than to develop an unfounded speculation.

Finally the discussion should focus on the toxicological significance of findings; after all, the purpose of the study is to study the toxicity of the test compound. No discussion at all is better than one which skirts around the issue of toxicity. Who is better placed than the author of the report to put findings into context? Always keep in mind that if you do not have the courage to put findings into a toxicological context, then someone else will!

4.6 The Conclusion

The golden rule in writing the Conclusion is that YOU SHOULD NOT JUMP TO CONCLUSIONS! The Conclusion of a toxicology report should put the results into perspective *with reference to the objective(s) of the study*. Therefore, the Conclusion of a toxicokinetic study should be restricted to toxicokinetic findings, the Conclusion of a study measuring bioequivalence of a new formulation should refer only to bioequivalence, the Conclusion of a study comparing target-organ toxicity in a test species with that of a reference species should be restricted to the principal results observed in the target organ investigated, etc.

Toxic dose levels as well as doses producing no toxic effects should always be identified. However, in studies on pharmaceutical compounds, the use of the terms "No-Effect Level", "No Observable Adverse Effect Level" and "No-Observable Effect Level" is often elusive, particularly if pharmacological effects are evident at the lowest dose level. Although these terms are not applicable to studies which reveal pharmacological effects at all dose levels, definition of a No-Effect Level is required by some regulations. Labels such as "toxicological no-effect level" or "dose level devoid of toxic effects" may be used. The target organ(s) for toxicity and/or the principal markers for toxicity should always be mentioned. The Conclusion of studies performed to determine suitable dose levels for subsequent investigations (e.g. sighting, maternal toxicity studies, range-finding or pre-carcinogenicity studies) should not include a dose level proposal for subsequent studies; new events may arise to change the perception of the data and hence dose proposal. However, if appropriate, the MTD (maximal tolerated dose) should be clearly identified.

In reproductive toxicology (e.g. embryofetal toxicity) studies, the Conclusion should attempt to relate maternal toxicity to fetal observations and identify the dose level at which no fetal or maternal effects were observed. The presence or absence of fetotoxic effects should always be stated. The Conclusion of maternal toxicity studies performed as range-finding studies for subsequent fetal-/embryo-toxicity studies should principally address maternally toxic dose levels. Fetal effects are of secondary interest in such studies and should therefore be interpreted conservatively.

In the interest of brevity and clarity, toxicological effects should be described qualitatively rather than quantitatively; this helps the reader to appreciate the importance of findings. If you cannot fit your "conclusions" into a few lines then you are probably rehashing your results. Sample Discussions and Conclusions are given in Examples 4.7 to 4.10.

Example 4.7   Discussion/Conclusion of a 1-month study in dogs

The maximal plasma drug concentrations of PP 27456 on day 3 were dose-related. Rapid clearance was observed at 20 mg/kg/day; the relatively lower clearance at 40 and 80 mg/kg/day resulted in a four- to ninefold increase in systemic drug exposure at these dose levels (when compared with the values noted at 20 mg/kg/day). This was most likely caused by saturation of metabolism and/or excretion. Consequently, PP 27456 accumulated at 40 and 80 mg/kg/day, resulting in markedly increased plasma drug concentrations on day 28, with corresponding AUC values which were four- and sevenfold higher than the respective values on day 3. This accumulation of the test compound may be responsible for the progressive appearance of adverse clinical signs observed at 40 and 80 mg/kg/day during the course of this study (progressive decrease in body weight gain and food consumption at 40 mg/kg/day, body weight loss and the progressive deterioration of clinical condition at 80 mg/kg/day).

A clear compound-related effect was evident at 80 mg/kg/day as shown by marked clinical signs, marked changes in clinical chemistry and hematology parameters, and histopathological changes in liver and bone marrow. Histo-pathologic evidence of hepatic centrilobular necrosis was associated with a marked increase in liver weight and accompanied by increased clinical chemistry markers (seven- to tenfold increases in alkaline phosphatase, ASAT and ALAT activities and plasma bilirubin values), and a four- to fivefold increase in hepatic microsomal cytochrome P450 content. Histopathologic evidence of hypocellular bone marrow was associated with a marked decrease in the principal RBC parameters. Additional histopathologic findings in the 80 mg/kg/day group, such as testicular atrophy, thymic and salivary gland atrophy and hypertrophy of the adrenal zona fasciculata, were possibly related to the poor condition of these

continued

animals, secondary to liver toxicity. The mild reductions in plasma electrolyte levels (chloride, calcium, potassium) at this dose level are likely to be related to PP 27567. The mechanism for these changes is unclear.

In contrast, administration of 40 mg/kg/day of PP 27456 produced no microscopically discernible changes in the liver. Induction (two- to threefold) of cytochrome P450, minimal to moderate increase in alkaline phosphatase and moderate increase in liver weights at this dose may be regarded as adaptive changes of the liver (Schulte-Hermann, 1972; Balazs *et al.*, 1978; Gopinath *et al.*, 1987).

At 20 mg/kg/day, a minimal (1.0– to 1.3-fold, compared with control mean values) increase of cytochrome P450 did not correlate with any other clinical chemistry variation or histopathologic changes. While the increase in cytochrome P450 may be regarded as a minimal adaptive effect of treatment, the values are well within our historical control range for this parameter, and were not considered toxicologically significant.

In conclusion, treatment of dogs for 30 days with oral doses of 80 mg/kg/day of PP 27456 produced toxicity of the liver and bone marrow. Findings at a dose level of 40 mg/kg/day were limited to adaptive changes in the liver. No evidence for adverse effects was observed at a dose level of 20 mg/kg/day of PP 27456.

Example 4.8   Discussion/Conclusion of a maternal toxicity study in rats

Signs of mild to moderate maternal toxicity (stained and soft feces, reduction in food intake and progressive body weight loss) were evident at 100 and 200 mg/kg. Therefore, the reduction in fetal and placental weights at these dose levels was considered to be related to the maternal effects at these doses. The delay in skeletal ossification observed at 200 mg/kg (increase in incidence of fetuses with three or four incomplete or unossified sternebral bones) was consistent with the lower fetal weight recorded at this dose level and was considered to be secondary to the maternal toxicity.

In conclusion, oral administration of PP 45678 to pregnant rats during the period of organogenesis at dose levels of 100 and 200 mg/kg/day produced maternal toxicity which was associated with reduced fetal and placental weights, and a reduction in skeletal ossification at 200 mg/kg/day. No evidence for adverse maternal or developmental effects was observed at a dose level of 50 mg/kg/day.

Example 4.9   Conclusion of a 1-month study in rats

In conclusion, single daily oral administration of PP 83211 to Sprague–Dawley rats for one month at dose levels of 0, 5, 25 and 125 mg/kg/day did not affect survival

---

continued

or hematologic parameters. A dose level of 125 mg/kg/day produced a mild reduction in mean body weight (−8% to −12%) and food consumption (−5% to −8%), moderate clinical signs (transient ataxia), a mild increase in ALAT and ASAT activity and a moderate increase in liver weight associated with centrilobular hypertrophy. Changes at 25 mg/kg were limited to a minimal increase in liver weight. No evidence of adverse effects was observed at 5 mg/kg/day.

Example 4.10   Conclusion of a carcinogenicity study in rats

The oral administration of PP 27567 to Sprague–Dawley rats at daily dose levels of 0, 2, 8 and 30 mg/kg/day for 24 months did not induce neoplastic or non-neoplastic histopathological changes. PP 27567 produced mainly effects consistent with its pharmacological activity. In addition, an increase in mean body weight as well as a decrease in mean survival in males treated at 8 and 30 mg/kg/day and in females receiving 30 mg/kg/day, were noted. In conclusion, no evidence of a carcinogenic potential was observed in this study and no indication for adverse effects was noted at a dose level of 2 mg/kg/day.

4.7 Final Thoughts

Writing a toxicology report is like all other human endeavors. Few, if any of us, are born with the innate skill to write clearly and concisely. These are skills which must be learned and honed through constant use, practice and self-criticism. Given the importance of the discovery of new and effective drugs for the well-being of mankind we have to ensure that potentially valuable new drugs are not lost through careless presentation of toxicology data. The most rigorously performed study is of little value if badly reported.

The golden rule for report writing is that there is no golden rule. It is the responsibility of the author(s) to do what is necessary to present data in the clearest and most comprehensible manner. If this requires going against established orthodoxy, then so be it!

5

Plasma Drug Concentrations (Toxicokinetic Data)

ROBERT J. SZOT

Consultant in Toxicology, Flemington, NJ, USA

The degree of systemic drug exposure determined by plasma drug concentrations provides a critical link for evaluating differences in toxicology between species and therefore in assessing the risk of human exposure. Exposure data are usually presented in a report as the toxicokinetic profile characterizing the concentration of the drug and/or its major metabolites in blood (plasma or serum) or other tissue over time. The toxicokinetic data serve as a surrogate of the dosage given to the animal and constitute a more accurate reference to a biological response than dosage. Thus the focus of the narrative of toxicokinetic data should be on its usefulness in evaluating toxicity data and not on simply describing the rate of change of drug concentration over time.

Toxicokinetic data should be reported as narrative and tables with minimal duplication of information between these two formats. The primary focus of the narrative is to provide qualitative information on systemic exposure relative to dosage and goals of the toxicity study. The tabular data should present the toxicokinetic data in a format in which details can be easily recognized and related to the narrative. The tabulated data should also help the writer to minimize the length of the narrative by avoiding sentences with long runs of numeric data. The use of graphic data should also be considered. Graphs can simplify complex relations or numerous data points between drug concentrations over time or between dosage groups.

The following reporting objectives should be considered in describing systemic drug exposure.

1   The degree of absorption of the compound using quantifying terms relative to expectations (e.g. poorly or well absorbed, if appropriate), dosage given (linear or saturation kinetics) and human blood concentrations (if known) should be described.

2   Differences in blood concentrations relative to sex and duration of dosing (evidence of accumulation or signs of metabolic induction) should be pointed out.

3   Exposure levels should be correlated with toxicity.

4 Always keep in mind any differences in dosing regimen (method, frequency, formulation) used in the toxicity study compared with that in humans.

5 Briefly describe blood collection methods, storage of samples prior to analysis and method of analysis.

When evaluating the degree of absorption, consideration should be given to drug effects that might have affected absorption. Emesis following oral dosing or severe local irritation following subcutaneous or intramuscular dosing could potentially alter the degree of systemic exposure. Take care that descriptions of absorption are appropriate to study conditions. Do not indicate that a compound given intravenously was "well absorbed".

Toxicokinetic data are usually reported in units of concentration (amount/volume) or area under the curve (AUC, amount.time/volume). When reporting concentrations, the same units should be used throughout the report and in all reports on the same compound. Consistency in units minimizes the chance of errors and maximizes readability and understanding of the report.

There is no correct degree of detail or format for writing any report. What is right depends on the laboratory's culture, history and study needs. However, the report narrative must always be reader-friendly and provide the necessary information to cover the study goals and to evaluate the data. Details can be tabulated in the appendix. Several reporting situations are provided in Examples 5.1–5.4.

Example 5.1

Methods

Concentrations of PP 27567 were measured in plasma collected from each dog at all dosage levels at 0.5, 1, 3 and 12 hours following dosing on dose days 1 and 89. Blood (approximately 1.5 ml) was collected from the jugular vein into a heparinized container. The plasma was stored at −10 °C prior to assay. The assay method consisted of extraction of drug from plasma into ethanol and analysis by high-pressure liquid chromatography (HPLC).

Results

PP 27567 was well absorbed following oral administration. Plasma concentrations were similar in males and were females and were generally dose-proportional. There was no evidence of self-induction of metabolism. Mean plasma concentrations at 1 hour (C_{max}) following the initial dose were 60, 120 and 600 μg/ml for males and 75, 135 and 550 μg/ml for females in the 3, 6 and 30 mg/kg/day dosage groups, respectively. Similar concentrations were observed on dose day 89. Mean AUCs (0–12 hours, combined data from both sexes) following the initial dose were 150, 240 and 845 μg.h/ml in the 3, 6 and 30 mg/kg/day dosage groups, respectively.

Example 5.2

Methods

Blood was collected from each monkey at 5, 15 and 30 minutes and 1, 3, 12 and 24 hours following intravenous dosing on dose days 1 and 28 for measurement of PP 27567 concentrations in plasma. At each interval approximately 0.5 ml of blood was collected into an EDTA-coated container. Following centrifugation, plasma samples were extracted on AASP C2 cartridges prior to separation by high-pressure liquid chromatography (HPLC).

Results

Plasma concentrations on dose day 28 are summarized in Table 5.1. Plasma concentrations and AUCs were dose-proportional on the first day of dosing and there were no apparent sex-related differences.

Table 5.1   PP 27567: 1-Month oral toxicity study in Cynomolgus monkeys – plasma concentrations on day 28.

Dose (mg/kg/day)	Sex[a]	Plasma concentration (range) μg/ml		AUC (mean value) μg.h/ml	
		0.25 h	24 h	AUC 0–7 h	AUC 0–24 h
10	M	2.5–3.6	nd[b]	21.2 ± 2.4	42.1 ± 4.5
	F	2.7–4.2	0.5–0.9	23.5 ± 2.7	44.7 ± 4.9
20	M	4.4–5.8	0.8–1.8	45.7 ± 5.4	92.8 ± 7.6
	F	3.2–6.7	0.9–2.3	46.9 ± 8.3	98.7 ± 9.8
80	M	18.9–21.3	16.5–18.4	164.3 ± 13.6	967.8 ± 56.9
	F	22.1–24.3	18.7–19.2	176.7 ± 18.5	987.2 ± 45.9

[a]Each value is the range or mean of 3 monkeys/sex.
[b]Concentration was below the limit of detection.

   PP 27567 was slowly, but completely eliminated by 24 hours following dosing with 10 or 20 mg/kg/day. Concentrations on day 1 were similar to those on day 28. However, at the 80 mg/kg/day dosage level, an approximate 4-fold increase in mean plasma concentration occurred on day 28. This datum indicates significant accumulation occurred at a dosage of 80 mg/kg/day. Systemic exposure in monkeys to daily dosages of 10 mg/kg was approximately twice that expected in humans given the therapeutic dosing regimen.

Discussion

Severe and persistent tremors with occasional convulsions were noted in all monkeys dosed with 80 mg/kg/day after the 20th dose day. These effects were probably associated with drug accumulation at this dosage level. Similar signs

---

continued

were not seen at lower dosages where accumulation was slight or did not occur. Accumulation probably resulted from a reduced rate of renal excretion resulting from the nephrotoxic effects of PP 27567 at this dosage level but not at lower levels. Reductions in urine excretion, increased urea nitrogen levels and tubular necrosis occurred at this dosage level. These observations are probably of no clinical significance since plasma concentrations at the proposed maximum clinical dose are approximately half those observed in monkeys dosed with 10 mg/kg/day.

Example 5.3

Methods

The systemic exposure of PP 27567 was measured in three satellite groups of 12 rats each. On dose days 1, 30 and 90, blood samples were collected from one rat/sex/group approximately 2, 6, 10 and 24 hours following subcutaneous dosing. Approximately 1.0 ml of blood was collected via the retro-orbital sinus (under CO_2 anesthesia) into glass tubes using no anticoagulants. Rats bled at each collection interval were euthanized by CO_2 asphyxiation and discarded. PP 27567 concentrations were determined by a radioimmunoassay procedure.

Results

Subcutaneously administered PP 27567 was well absorbed in a dose-proportional manner with no apparent difference between sexes. Peak plasma concentrations occurred approximately 6 hours post-dosing. At 24 hours post-dosing on dose day 1, PP 27567 was detected only in rats dosed with 10 and 30 mg/kg/day. On dose day 1, peak plasma concentrations were 4, 10 and 27 μg/ml as opposed to concentrations at 24 hours of 0, 4 and 13 μg/ml for the 3, 10 and 30 mg/kg/day dosage groups, respectively. The graphs below show that, as the study progressed, plasma concentrations of PP 27567 decreased. At the end of the study (day 90), plasma concentrations of PP 27567 in rats dosed with 30 mg/kg were approximately one-third of those measured on the first dose day. (See Figures 5.1–5.3.)

Discussion

The decrease in plasma concentrations of PP 27567 over the course of dosing suggests that self-induction of hepatic metabolism had occurred. This is consistent with the dose-proportional increases in liver weight and proliferation of the smooth endoplasmic reticulum observed by electronmicroscopy of liver tissues. The reduction in plasma concentrations over time accounts for the decrease in clinical signs observed during this study.

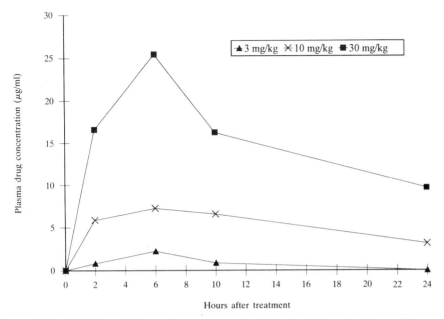

Figure 5.1 PP 27567: 90-Day subcutaneous toxicity study in rats. Mean plasma drug concentrations (µg/ml) on day 1 (male and female values combined)

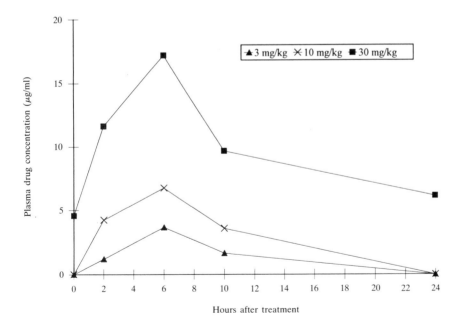

Figure 5.2 PP 27567: 90-Day subcutaneous toxicity study in rats. Mean plasma drug concentrations (µg/ml) on day 30 (male and female values combined)

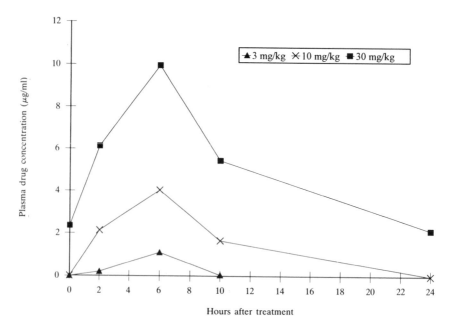

Figure 5.3 PP 27567: 90-Day subcutaneous toxicity study in rats. Mean plasma drug concentrations (μg/ml) on day 90 (male and female values combined)

Example 5.4

Methods

Blood samples were collected approximately 2 hours after dosing from the first 6 rabbits per group that survived on gestation days 7 and 19 (dose days 1 and 13). The blood was collected from the medial artery in the ear and immediately transferred into heparinized tubes. On gestation day 19, one dam per dosage group underwent caesarean section approximately 0.5 hours following dosing, and fetuses were removed. Blood was collected by decapitation under CO_2 anesthesia and pooled for each litter. Plasma from the dams and fetuses was stored at $-20°C$. Concentrations of parent drug (PP 27567) and its major metabolite (PP 39876) were determined by reversed phase HPLC. Two other metabolites (PP 39877 and PP 39878) of PP 27567 were not measured, because they were present at less than 2% of the total level of parent drug and metabolites that could be detected.

Results

At 2 hours post-dosing, plasma concentrations of PP 27567 and its major metabolite (PP 39876) in pregnant rabbits appeared to increase in a dose-dependent manner on both gestation days 7 and 19. Marginal increases in concentrations of PP 27567 occurred during the dosing period. Plasma levels

continued

of the parent drug and its metabolite in the pregnant animals are given in Table 5.2.

Table 5.2. PP 27567: Maternal toxicity study in pregnant rabbits – plasma drug concentrations 2 hours after treatment.

| Dose (mg/kg/day) | Day[a] | Plasma concentrations (μg/ml)[b] | |
		PP 27567 (parent drug)	PP 39876 (metabolite)
10	1	0.4 ± 0.1	7.6 ± 4.3
	13	0.5 ± 0.8	13.2 ± 2.9
20	1	1.1 ± 0.2	17.2 ± 5.4
	13	0.9 ± 0.2	31.3 ± 13.7
30	1	1.7 ± 0.3	22.1 ± 7.5
	13	1.1 ± 0.4	35.6 ± 27.7
40	1	1.9 ± 0.5	29.0 ± 11.3
	13	1.8 ± 0.7	64.6 ± 28.6

[a]Correspond to gestation days 7 and 19.
[b]Mean $\pm$ standard deviation of 6 rabbits/dose group.

Fetal exposure at the end of the dosing period was limited to the metabolite PP 39876 at the 30 ($2.5 \pm 1.7 \mu$g/ml) and 40 ($4.7 \pm 2.6 \mu$g/ml) mg/kg dosage levels only. No metabolite was detected at lower dosages. Parent drug was not detected in fetal plasma at any dosage level.

Discussion

Exposure to PP 27567 and PP 39876 in pregnant rabbits was dose dependent and ranged from approximately one-half to twice that expected in humans given the therapeutic dosage. This is in contrast to exposure to metabolite, which appears to range from two- to fourfold greater than that expected in humans. The data suggest that the rate of metabolism of parent drug may be greater in the rabbit than human. The relatively small difference in maternal concentrations between the 30 and 40 mg/kg dosages and the significant degree in maternal toxicity observed at these dosages suggest that the metabolite may be more toxic than the parent drug. Similarly, fetal deaths were observed only at those dosage levels (30 and 40 mg/kg/day) at which the metabolite was detected in the fetuses.

6

Reporting In-life Observations and Measurements

G. J. NOHYNEK

Rhône-Poulenc Rorer, Vitry sur Seine, France

The results of in-life observations/measurements of *in vivo* toxicity studies are commonly described in the following order:

1   mortality
2   clinical signs and observations
3   body weight evaluations
4   food consumption data
5   other in-life evaluations, e.g. cardiovascular measurements.

6.1 Mortality

Mortality is the most serious result of toxicity and must be described with great care. Describe mortality with reference to animals and/or dose identification, time of death and clinical observations associated with or prior to death. Whenever mortality occurs in a toxicology study, it must be clearly distinguished as compound-related, procedure-related or caused by other factors. The incidence of mortality and dose identification should always be *numerical*, e.g. "5/20 males died at *150* mg/kg". Necropsy observations should not be included in this section except to explain non-compound-related death, e.g. unscheduled or accidental death resulting from gavage error.

   A description of mortality which occurred in satellite groups which were used for plasma drug determination may be included in this section if death is considered to be related to the compound and not to blood sampling procedures. Mortality caused by accidents (gavage accidents, accidents during handling or restraining of animals) should be described separately, including clinical signs preceding death and/or the evidence (e.g. necropsy findings) for classifying these deaths as accidental. Example: "Two animals [male No. 304 (40 mg/kg) and female No. 605 (80 mg/kg)] were found dead on days 15 and 22, respectively. Necropsy findings in these animals (congested lungs, traces of white particles in the bronchi) suggest that their deaths were due to gavage accident". If a high incidence of mortality occurs in a study, and particularly if compound-related mortality occurs concurrently with mortality not related to the test compound, use a table to improve comprehensibility (see Examples 6.1 and 6.2).

Sacrifice for ethical reasons should be addressed in this section; include a brief description of the rationale for sacrifice, e.g. "Male 41 (24 mg/kg) was found in a moribund condition on day 21 and was sacrificed", or "Two males at 50 mg/kg displayed severe clinical signs (severe ataxia, convulsions) and were sacrificed for

Example 6.1   Use of table to report mortality details in a single-dose study

Table 6.1 PP 27567: Single-dose oral study in mice – incidence of mortality.

Dose (mg/kg)	Control	50	250	500
Males	0/5	1/50	3/5	5/5
Females	1/5 [a]	0/5	1/5	3/5

[a]attributed to accidental death of female F 55 (gavage error – see necropsy findings).

Example 6.2   Use of table to report mortality details in a repeated-dose study

Four animals died during the course of the study as described in Table 6.2.

Table 6.2 PP 27567: 1-Month repeated-dose oral toxicity in rats – mortality.

Animal number	Group/dose	Signs/day of death
M 106	Control	Reduced motor activity, dyspnea from day 16; found dead on day 17
F 613	50 mg/kg	Died during blood sampling on day 14
M 408	500 mg/kg	Day 23: nasal discharge containing blood; sacrificed on day 24
F 915	500 mg/kg	Day 26: dyspnea within minutes after compound administration, followed by death

Based on the circumstances of these deaths and/or necropsy findings (e.g. congested lungs, traces of white particles in the bronchi) they were considered to be accidental (due to gavage error for animals M106, M408 and F915, or due to the anesthesia and/or blood-sampling procedures for F613).

ethical reasons". However, avoid referring to mortality of animals sacrificed for ethical reasons as "*compound-related*" mortality! However, you may say: "Mortality (*including sacrifice of moribund animals for ethical reasons*) was 0/10, 2/10 and 6/10 at 2, 8 and 32 mg/kg, respectively".

In those reproductive toxicology studies which had a high incidence of mortality and sacrifice due to ethical reasons, a table explaining the incidence of unscheduled death, animals sacrificed following abortion or sacrificed for ethical reasons may be included (see Example 6.3).

Example 6.3   Use of table to report mortality details in a reproductive toxicity study

One animal at 300 mg/kg/day was found dead on day 16 of the study. On days 18 and 19, 6/19, 1/20 and 1/20 animals in the 300 mg/kg/day, 100 mg/kg/day and control groups, respectively, were sacrificed following abortion. In addition, 2 animals at 300 mg/kg/day and 1 animal at 100 mg/kg/day were found moribund and sacrificed on days 17 and 18. No mortality occurred at 30 mg/kg/day. The incidence of mortality is shown in Table 6.3.

Table 6.3 PP 27567: Maternal toxicity study in rabbits - mortality.

Dose group	Control	30 mg/kg/day	100 mg/kg/day	300 mg/kg/day
Found dead	0	0	0	1
Sacrificed (ethical)	0	0	1	2
Sacrificed (abortion)	1	0	1	6
Total	1/20	0/20	2/20	9/20

6.2 Clinical Signs and Observations

This section should first describe compound-induced symptomatic or behavioral changes (ataxia, emesis, mydriasis, absence of motor activity, etc.), followed by observations or signs related to general appearance (alopecia, stained fur, etc.). The incidence of clinical signs should be numerical, if possible. The description of clinical signs should include (numerical) data about their onset, duration, incidence and intensity. The severity of a clinical sign may be graded mild, moderate, or marked/severe. However, grading scales of clinical signs should only be used in exceptional cases. Avoid using more than three severity grades. If grading scales are used, the grading should be defined in the text or using a footnote of a table. The terminology used for an individual sign should correspond to a clinical sign dictionary or the respective Standard Operation Procedure. Signs and symptoms should preferably be descriptive, using simple terminology and avoiding diagnostic terms, terms which are poorly defined or not commonly used in toxicology (see attached list). Rare clinical signs which require use of the appropriate medical or veterinarian terminology should be defined and, if necessary, explained in the text when used for the first time. Examples:

- "Paresis (*weakness*) of the hind limbs was observed on day 12 in one animal (F707, 80 mg/kg). This sign became increasingly severe during days 13 to 15, warranting sacrifice for ethical reasons on day 16."
- "Opisthotonos (*prolonged and severe muscle spasm of the back causing arching of the back, backbending of the head with rigid, extended limbs*) was noted on day 2 in two male dogs (M205, F707) in the 80 mg/kg group."

Sporadic clinical signs which are not related to the compound but which appear in the tables of the individual clinical observations in the appendix of the report should be addressed and dismissed (if not compound-related) in a final phrase of this section. A table may be used to aid comprehension of multiple clinical signs (see Example 6.5). In reproductive toxicology reports, the incidence of abortion may be described in this section.

6.3 A Clinical Signs Glossary

The following is an example of a simple list of clinical signs which is by no means complete. However, it is more practical to use a simple list which includes only the *most common* clinical signs. This prevents overloading your laboratory's glossary with diagnostic terms and potential misuse of terminology. Diagnostic terms for rare clinical signs should be defined on a case-by-case basis after a careful examination of the affected animal(s).

General appearance and condition

Abortion
Agalactorrhea
Alopecia
Arched back
Broken teeth
Brown stains on muzzle
Cold to the touch
Cough
Discoloration of mucous membranes
Discoloration of the skin (site, color)
Discolored haircoat (color)
Distended abdomen
Excessive salivation
Galactorrhea
Hunched back
Increased firmness (site)
Loss of teeth
Mass (site)

Nasal discharge
Pale skin (site)
Piloerection
Reduced elasticity of the skin
Rough hair coat
Scab (site, size, appearance)
Skin flakes
Soiled ano-genital area
Soiled fur
Stained teeth
Swelling (site)
Tail loss (partial/complete)
Thin body
Thin hair coat
Umbilical hernia
Vulvar discharge
Wet fur
Wound (site, size, appearance)

Eyes

Destruction of eye
Dry eye
Eye opacity
Eyelids (partially) closed
Lacrimation
Mydriasis

Pinpoint pupils
Protruding eye
Protrusion of nictitating membrane
Red area around eye
Red conjunctiva
Sunken eye

Functions

Absence of urine
Absent/reduced feces
Discolored feces (color)
Discolored urine (color)
Hiccup
Increased/decreased respiration rate
Increased/decreased water intake
Labored respiration

Liquid feces
Noisy respiration
Reduced/increased urine volume
Regurgitation
Retching
Soft feces
Vomiting

Behavior

Aggression
Agitation
Chewing
Circling movements
Head tilt
Hyperreactive to external stimuli

Hyporeactive to external stimuli
Licking
Lying on the cage floor
Unresponsive to external stimuli
Vocalization

Activity/Movements

Absence of motor activity
Convulsions
Decreased motor activity
Flaccidity of limbs
Incoordination
Increased motor activity

Lameness of limbs
Loss of righting reflex
Loss of use of limbs
Rigidity of limbs
Tremors

Example 6.4   Clinical signs

Treatment-related signs occurred from week 2 through study termination: all animals treated with 150 mg/kg/day and 3/4 male animals at 50 mg/kg/day displayed dryness of the nose and redness of the bulbar conjunctivae. In addition, all animals at 50 and 150 mg/kg/day, and 3/4 males at 15 mg/kg/day had mydriasis.

53

continued

All signs appeared within 15 minutes after administration of PP 27456 and persisted approximately 6 to 8 hours. All other clinical signs recorded during this study are commonly observed in our laboratory and were not considered to be related to PP 27456.

Example 6.5 Table of clinical signs

Clinical signs (reduced motor activity and dyspnea) were observed throughout the study with dose-related incidence, severity and duration, and appeared within 10 minutes following treatment. Their incidence, severity and duration are summarized in Table 6.4.

Table 6.4 PP 27567: Single oral toxicity in rats – clinical signs.

Dose (mg/kg)	Observation	Incidence (daily)	Severity	Duration
5	reduced motor activity[a]	M: 3/10 F: 0/10	mild	0.5 to 2 hours
20	reduced motor activity	M: 7/10 F: 2/10	moderate mild	1 to 1.5 hours 0.5 to 1 hour
	dyspnea[b]	M: 1/10	mild	1 to 2 minutes
80	reduced motor activity	M: 10/10 F: 6/10	marked moderate	8 to 24 hours 2 to 4 hours
	dyspnea	M: 8/10 F: 4/10	marked mild	10 to 25 minutes 5 to 10 minutes

[a]Reduced motor activity: mild – sluggishness of animals; moderate – sleepy animals/reduced reaction to external stimuli; marked – absence of reaction to external stimuli, animals asleep for > 2 hours following treatment.
[b]Dyspnea: mild – occasional gasping; moderate – 1–2 times per minute; marked – episodes of continuous gasping lasting more than 1 minute, followed by brief recovery and reoccurrence.

6.4 Abortions (Rabbit Segment II/Embryofetal Development Toxicity Studies)

Strictly speaking, abortions represent a clinical sign and should be reported under this section. On the other hand, since animals having aborted are normally sacrificed for ethical reasons, the incidence of abortions may also be reported within the mortality section, or within a separate section. However, in my view, abortions are preferably reported within the Clinical Signs and Observations section of rabbit Segment II studies.

Example 6.6   Compound-related abortions

Six females in the 300 mg/kg/day group, one female in the 100 mg/kg/day group and one control female aborted during the treatment period. The pregnancy losses of five of the 300 mg/kg/day females were preceded by body weight loss, reduced food intake and reduced fecal output; the sixth female had no significant history. It is known that adverse treatment, including dietary deprivation (Matsuzawa *et al.*, 1983), can lead to abortion in rabbits. Thus, all of the abortions observed in this study can be considered to be related to changes in maternal status, with PP 27567-related maternal toxicity contributing to the increased incidence of abortion when the drug was administered at 300 mg/kg/day.

Example 6.7   Abortions not related to the test compound

One control female, two females in the 30 mg/kg/day group and one female in the 300 mg/kg/day group aborted during the study. In view of the group distribution and the absence of a treatment-relationship, involvement of PP 27567 was considered unlikely.

6.5 Body Weight Data

Describe body weight changes relative to dose and sex. As a rule, descriptions of body weight changes refer to group mean changes for rodents and rabbits, and individual animal change for large animals, i.e. dogs and monkeys. With two different control groups, e.g. in intravenous studies which include a vehicle control and a saline control group, group mean body weight changes in treated groups should always be related to vehicle control group means. Body weight changes in large animals may be related to the control group or to individual body weights at study initiation. Be clear of your meaning when expressing *changes in body weight* versus *changes in body weight gain*. Generally, it is simpler not to attempt to describe a lower mean body weight *gain*, but instead to refer to *lower group mean body weights* in treated groups at study termination or at interim weighing points. Whenever there are multiple changes in body weight across treated groups, they may be described using a table (see Example 6.9).

Please note that the term "body weight" is generally used in the singular unless one refers to several groups or specifically to several animals, e.g. "Body weight in the group receiving 74 mg/kg/day was unaffected. There was no compound-related change in body weight in the groups receiving 75 or 150 mg/kg PP 46567." *But*: "5/10 animals receiving 55 mg/kg/day had lower body weights".

Example 6.8   Body weight data

PP 27567 produced dose- and compound-related effects on body weight: on day 29, males treated with 100 and 300 mg/kg/day had a lower mean body weight (-8% and -12%, when compared with control values); in females, the respective mean body weight differences on day 29 at 100 and 300 mg/kg/day were -11% and -16%, respectively. The difference in body weight was statistically significant at 300 mg/kg/day for both male and female groups. No effect on body weight was observed in the groups receiving 30 mg/kg/day.

Example 6.9   Body weight table

Table 6.5 PP 27567: 6-Month repeated dose toxicity in rats – mean body weight on days 62, 127 and 182 of the study (percentage change compared with control mean values).

Dose (mg/kg/day)	Sex	Day 62	Day 127	Day 182
5	M	nc[a]	nc	-3
	F	nc	-2	-6^*
25	M	nc	-5	-9^*
	F	-5	-8^*	-12^*
75	M	-9^*	-12^*	-17^*
	F	-12^*	-19^*	$-^b$

$^*p<0.05$
[a] no change
[b] treatment discontinued on day 128

6.6 Food Consumption

Describe food consumption changes according to sex and dose. Whenever multiple changes across several treated groups are observed, they should be described in a table. Minor or elementary changes may be described in the text. Changes may be expressed as percentage change compared with control means for rodents and rabbits. For dogs or primates, food consumption in treated groups may be compared with control means with sufficient group size and body weight homogeneity. However, food consumption in dogs is generally described semi-quantitatively. In short-term studies (<1 month) in large animals, food consumption may be compared with pre-study mean and/or individual values. Correlate changes in food consumption with corresponding changes in body weight. Please note that the term "food consumption" is always used in the singular!

Example 6.10 Food consumption – rodents

In all treated groups, PP 27567 produced a compound- and dose-related decrease in food consumption as shown in Table 6.6.

Table 6.6 PP 27567: 28-Day repeated dose oral toxicity in rats – food consumption during week 4 (percentage change compared with control mean values).

Dose (mg/kg/day)	Males	Females
30	−2	−4
100	−9*	−12*
300	−15*	−19*

*$p < 0.05$ (comparison of means with respective control means)

The decreased food consumption in males at 100 and 300 mg/kg/day was statistically significant and correlated to the lower body weight gain observed at these dose levels. While a relation to treatment of the lower food consumption at 30 mg/kg/day cannot be excluded, this change was minimal, within the range of the common variation of this parameter, and is therefore considered to be of no toxicological significance.

Example 6.11 Food consumption – dogs

Food consumption of dogs receiving 100 mg/kg/day was severely decreased (approximately −75% in females and −50% in males). At 30 mg/kg/day, a sporadic decrease in food consumption was noted with a slightly higher incidence in females than in males, while at 10 mg/kg/day food consumption was unaffected by treatment. The lower food consumption at 100 mg/kg/day correlated with the observed body weight loss in males and females.

Example 6.12 Food consumption – rabbits

1 Food intake of 45 and 150 mg/kg/day females was decreased during the second half of the treatment period and correlated with the lower body weight gain in these groups. Food consumption of females in the 15 mg/kg/day group was unaffected by treatment.

2 A dose-related and statistically significant decrease in food consumption was recorded in all treated groups for the dosing period. Following the recovery period, food intake was similar in all groups.

6.7 Cardiovascular Parameters

6.7.1 *Electrocardiography*

Cardiovascular parameters are of particular interest as potential markers in clinical trials. However, care should be taken with respect to the meaning of the individual parameters in the human clinical situation when addressing changes in canine ECGs (e.g. "sinus arrhythmia" is pathologic in man but "respiratory sinus arrhythmia" is physiologic in dogs). Always report the quantitative change (are there any modifications in parameters or values?) before the qualitative ones (are there any rhythm abnormalities?). For quantitative analysis, describe the changes numerically. Complex and multiple changes should be reported using a table.

Example 6.13 Cardiovascular parameters not modified

> Heart rate values, PR, QRS and QT duration were not modified by PP 27567. No treatment-related changes in rhythm were noted.

Example 6.14 Increase in heart rate

> Two hours following administration of PP 27567, animals treated at 200 mg/kg had increased heart rates (20–30% when compared with pre-test values) and a concomitant reduction in QT interval (−12% to −15%, when compared with pre-test values). These changes were no longer present 24 hours after treatment. PQ and QRS interval were not modified by the treatment.

Example 6.15 Changes in ECG parameters

> In week 4, monomorph interpolated ventricular premature beats and a transient bundle branch block were noted in the ECG of one male dog (M31) treated at 100 mg/kg/day. These changes were neither observed in ECGs performed 24 hours later, nor in those performed at week 13. Ventricular premature beats and bundle branch block may occur spontaneously in dogs (Patterson *et al.*, 1961); since these changes were observed only in a single examination in one animal, they were considered to be of spontaneous origin and not to be related to administration of PP 27567.

Example 6.16 Increase in heart rates – table

> Heart rates measured during the pre-test period and during the study before the administration of PP 27567 were comparable in all groups (range: 85–134/min). During the treatment period, a dose-related increase in heart rate was noted in all treated groups 1 to 2 hours after treatment. This is shown in Table 6.7.

continued

Table 6.7 PP 27567: 1-Month oral toxicity study in dogs. Range of heart rates (and percentage mean increase, compared with pre-administration group mean values) 1 to 2 hours after administration of PP 27567 on days 5, 35, and 150 of the study.

Group/dose (mg/kg)	Day 5	Day 35	Day 150
Control	88–123	67–112	65–89
0.2	112–165 (+30%)	105–145 (+28%)	103–154 (+25%)
0.4	132–188 (+45%)	138–193 (+51%)	142–195 (+55%)
0.8	176–223 (+76%)	186–221 (+71%)	170–213 (+65%)

Heart rates in all groups taken 24 hours after treatment with PP 27567 were comparable to control or pre-test values.

6.7.2 Systolic Blood Pressure

In standard toxicology studies on non-rodents, both systolic and diastolic pressure are generally measured, although the evaluation is principally performed using the systolic arterial pressure.

Example 6.17   Blood pressure not affected by treatment

The values of systolic and diastolic blood pressure were not affected by treatment.

Example 6.18   Compound-related change in blood pressure

A compound-related increase in blood pressure was measured in the groups receiving 60 and 120 mg/kg/day on day 21, approximately 2 h following administration of PP 27567. In 60 mg/kg females, the mean systolic arterial pressure increased by about 20%, when compared with pre-test values. In the 120 mg/kg group, the corresponding increases were +20% in males and +32% in females. No compound-related effect was measured at 30 mg/kg. Twenty-four hours after treatment, arterial blood pressure was comparable in all groups.

Example 6.19   Use of a table for blood pressure values

A dose-related reduction in mean systolic blood pressure was noted 1 to 2 hours after treatment in all treated groups, relative to pre-treatment values. The extent

continued

of this effect was comparable on days 5, 55 and 150 of the study and is shown in Table 6.8.

Table 6.8   PP 27567: 6-Month oral toxicity in dogs – change of mean systolic blood pressure, compared with pre-treatment group mean values. Values on study days 5, 55 and 150, 1 to 2 hours after administration of PP 27567.

Group (mg/kg/day)	Day 5	Day 55	Day 150
Control	+3.8 mm	+5.5 mm	+6.8 mm
0.5	−26.0 mm	−31.3 mm	−19.3 mm
1.0	−40.0 mm	−46.2 mm	−34.7 mm
2.0	−56.4 mm	−55.2 mm	−9.7 mm

Systolic blood pressure values, taken 24 hours after administration of PP 27567 were comparable to control or pre-test values.

6.8 Ophthalmology

Describe all compound-related changes first and indicate the number of animals/sex/dose with the change.

Example 6.20   Ophthalmic observations

All lesions observed were considered typical for the age and strain of animals examined. There were no findings of toxicological significance.

A bilateral hypopigmentation of the fundus was observed in one control male at all examinations. A slight unilateral focal posterior lens opacity was noted in one 100 mg/kg/day female in week 13. The latter finding is commonly observed in dogs of this strain and age and was therefore not considered to be related to treatment. The main ocular findings were either of embryological origin (remnants of hyaloid vessels) or variations on the aspects of the vessels of the bulbar conjunctiva. The latter observation remained within physiological limits and is commonly observed in dogs of this age and provenance.

Example 6.21   Ophthalmic observations

Remnants of hyaloid vessels or a noticeable suture line of the anterior cortex of the lens were observed during the pre-study examination and on day 30 in some control animals and in some animals at 125 mg/kg/day. These vestigial fetal structures were no longer observed at the end of the study and were attributed to the young age of the animals. Small opalescent vesicles were observed in the

continued

superficial part of the corneal stroma in some male animals of the control, the 125 mg/kg/day and 5 mg/kg/day groups. This lesion was diagnosed as corneal dystrophy. Some minor changes were noted in the nucleus of the lens in animals from the control, 5 and 25 mg/kg/day groups. A comparable incidence of these lesions has been reported for Sprague-Dawley rats of this strain and age (Taradach and Greaves, 1984). In absence of the dose-relationship and since the incidence of these changes remained within our historical control values for incidence for these lesions, these changes were considered to be of spontaneous origin.

Reporting Clinical Pathology Results

M. Y. WELLS

Rhône-Poulenc Rorer, Drug Safety Department, Vitry sur Seine, France

and S. GOSSELIN

ITR Laboratories Canada Inc., Montreal, Canada

7.1 A Few Words on Data Evaluation

Hematology, clinical chemistry and urinalysis data can be among the most difficult data within a given study to evaluate, interpret and report. While the guidelines on how to write this section should give you some ideas on how to evaluate data, there is significant information on this subject that cannot be obtained herein. Also, because complete and thoughtful assessment of these data can be a trying process even for those specifically trained in clinical pathology, and because so many of us who must work with it are *not* trained in this area, a few words on the philosophy of data evaluation seem to be in order.

Methods of clinical pathology data evaluation include the use of statistics and the comparison of data from treated animals with absolute control, vehicle control, pretest, and/or historical control values. The method(s) chosen can vary with the species used and the length of study performed. Correlation between clinical pathology, in-life observations and anatomic pathology data is highly desirable but often not possible, and thus there is often no additional support for the conclusions drawn from analysis of clinical pathology data. Moreover, clinical pathology parameters are presumably more sensitive than histopathology for the interpretation of some toxicologically significant effects, which accentuates the importance of their accurate interpretation.

Statistics are often used for the assessment of clinical pathology data; but reliance on this type of evaluation alone often leads to the erroneous attribution of toxicological significance to "flagged" data, as well as erroneous inattention to data which are far more important for the interpretation of compound-related effects. For example, a large standard deviation can cause a compound-treated group to appear statistically similar to its control group, even when one or several individual values in the treatment group do not fall within the control range. Closer evaluation of these individual values may reveal a compound-related effect. On the other hand, statistically significant values may be within the range of normal variation; these should be minimized or dismissed when writing the clinical pathology report. Thus, statistics should be *neither the sole nor the primary* criteria for determining the toxicological significance of clinical pathology findings.

Among the species used in industrial toxicology safety assessment, large animals (e.g. dogs, monkeys, rabbits) generate the data which are the most complicated to evaluate. The number of animals per group is often less than five, meaning that the power of statistical analysis is significantly reduced. The wide range of individual variation in these animals requires more rigorous assessment of the data they generate, which should include evaluation of raw data from each individual animal. In these situations, individual animal data may take precedence over mean values.

All data should be evaluated and reported in relation to study controls. These are generally animals given the vehicle only. When two control groups are used (e.g. saline and vehicle control groups in intravenous studies), any differences between the vehicle and absolute control groups should be reported. The values from compound-treated groups should be compared with those of the vehicle control group to identify potential compound-related effects. When treated animals have laboratory values outside the study control range, historical control and pretest data (when available) may be evaluated to gain perspective on the significance of the observed variations. This does not mean that comparisons to pretest or historical control data must be reported; these are mentioned in the report only if they cause you to doubt or alter your interpretation of values in treated groups as compared with study controls.

In large animal studies, pretest analyses are usually performed, while in small animal (primarily rodent) studies, they are rarely performed. Pretest data should be considered in the overall evaluation of data for large animal studies of a duration of three months or less. In studies where animals are to be handled extensively and/or repeatedly bled, two to three pretest bleeds provide a more reliable database. In many, cases however, such an extensive base is not available. For longer studies, the age difference in the animals between study onset and study termination makes pretest data less useful in assessing compound-related changes (this may be less true in monkey studies if the animals are mature at the time of study initiation).

In the pretest period, animals destined for compound administration should be evaluated in relation to pretest control animals to discern whether or not any differences among these groups are appreciable before study initiation. During the study and at its termination, treatment values from individual animals in each group should be compared with their respective values during the pretreatment phase, so that each animal serves as its own control. Additionally, values from individual animals in a specific group may be compared with the range of values observed in that pretreatment group (e.g. values from high-dose animals should be compared with those of pretest "high-dose" animals, and not those from pretest control animals).

Pretest values from all groups may be used to form one large pretest reference range, but *only if* there are no differences observed among the pretest groups. This is not usually necessary, but may be desirable if the number of animals per group is very small.

Historical control data are another source of information which can be used to evaluate clinical pathology parameters. Many clinical pathologists limit their use of this database to the evaluation of animals during the acclimatization period because they believe that historical control values are too broad and not representative enough of the animals on study. For evaluation of changes occurring during studies using large animals, many favor pretest data over historical control data.

When historical controls are used during a study, they must be matched with the evaluated study parameters by age and by sex. Just as pretest data are not especially useful for parameters evaluated 6 months after study initiation, a historical control database for animals aged 6 months will not be very useful for interpreting data obtained from animals aged 14 months.

Differences in mean or individual values between treated and control groups which are determined to be compound-related may fall into the historical control and/or pretest range. If you believe that the observed changes are not biologically significant, then you may refer to these databases to support your position. However, if you do believe the changes to be significant, the fact that the values fall within reference ranges should not alter your conclusion. In other words, it is irresponsible to summarily dismiss compound-related effects simply because their values fall within reference range.

In rodent studies, the range of individual variation in clinical pathology parameters is smaller, and concurrent study controls are likely to constitute a sufficient database with which to compare and evaluate changes in treated animals. This is generally true regardless of the length of the study performed. However, in studies longer than 52 weeks, it is important to realize that data from all groups (including controls) are increasingly subject to variations secondary to age-related changes. In the combined chronic toxicity/carcinogenicity studies performed in the chemical industry for example, clinical pathology parameters are evaluated periodically through the entire study, which usually lasts 104 weeks. The data collected after 52 weeks generally yield little useful information with regard to primary compound-related effects, because age-related renal disease and spontaneous tumor generation become more prevalent, beginning at this time. These pathological changes affect clinical pathology parameters, and are likely to complicate the interpretation of any effects resulting directly from compound administration. Thus, if you are forced to interpret data in a study such as this, be fully aware of the "background noise" with which you are dealing.

The end result of the data evaluation described above should be the determination of all changes resulting from compound administration. In addition to the comparison of data with one or more reference ranges, the presence of a dose-relationship and/or the reversibility of an effect help to determine whether or not variations are compound-related. These issues are further described in the next section of this chapter.

While this preface in no way pretends to offer the reader a crash course in the evaluation of clinical pathology data, we hope that it highlights some general principles and, perhaps more importantly, some pitfalls of data interpretation in this domain. Before going on to the section addressing the actual writing of a clinical pathology report, here is a final note of caution: *avoid overinterpretation of data but beware of under-reporting effects because of data which are overlooked!*

7.2 Reporting the Data

As in all types of writing, clarity of expression is paramount in producing a high-quality document. It is equally important to keep in mind the final audience for whom you are writing (e.g. the regulatory authorities who will ultimately pass judgment on the compound being assessed, the physicians who will use your conclusions to plan clinical trials), and to prepare your report in a way that will be the most comprehensible for that audience. Finally, make every attempt to express your findings succinctly, without sacrificing necessary information which could compromise the reader's understanding of the conclusions presented.

You want to focus the reader's attention on what you believe to be important. Therefore, limit the scope of your descriptions of secondary and incidental changes so that you do not require paragraphs of text to explain them. The meat of the report should address compound-related changes.

Regardless of the number of databases (study controls, historical controls, etc.) used to evaluate studies, data are usually reported in relation to study control values. Additional information regarding data reviewed in relation to pretest and/or historical control values should be included when it helps clarify study results. An example of such a situation would be the following: "Minimal increases in phosphorus excretion were observed in males and females (+20% and +30% of mean control values, respectively) at 120 mg/kg/day. These values were increased over pretest values, but were within the range of historical control data. Thus they were not considered to be biologically significant".

Whether one is reporting hematology, clinical chemistry, or urinalysis values, answering the following questions will ensure complete reporting of the information required in this (or any) section of a toxicology report.

7.2.1 Are There Compound-related Changes?

The most important information given in any section of a toxicology report is whether or not there are effects related to compound administration. The first paragraph of the section should address this question. If there are no compound-related changes, simply state that none was observed; but if compound-related changes are present, they must be specifically identified. State the numeric dose levels at which the effects were noted, and whether one or both sexes were affected. If the number of changes is small, you may indicate their magnitude and direction in this paragraph as well. Identify any effects which have statistical significance (remember that statistical significance alone does not mean that an effect is compound-related!). See Example 7.1.

Example 7.1

> The administration of PP 19875 was associated with a moderate, statistically significant increase in ALAT (fivefold increase over mean control values) at 100 mg/kg in males only.

If there is only one effect, it can be fully described in the opening paragraph. If there are several changes to describe, you may summarize them in the opening statement and quantify them in subsequent paragraphs. Alternatively, you may choose to provide a list of the changes in the opening paragraph (see Example 7.2).

Example 7.2

Compound-related clinical chemistry findings (as compared with mean vehicle control values) consisted of:

- a mild increase in ALAT at 100 mg/kg (+80%)
- a mild decrease in triglycerides at 50 and 100 mg/kg (not less than −35%)
- a moderate increase in cholesterol at 25, 50 and 100 mg/kg (not greater than +45%)
- a moderate dose-related increase in BUN at 25, 50 and 100 mg/kg (+10%, +35% and +50%, respectively).

Large amounts of data or otherwise complicated data are best reported in the form of tables, figures and/or graphs. When using tables, values which are statistically significant should be indicated; these are more easily visualized in the tabular format than in prose.

Once you have made your opening statement, elaborate the results supporting that statement. Group related effects in a single paragraph (e.g. changes in liver enzymes, cholesterol and triglycerides indicate an effect on the liver and should be discussed together). Some clinical pathologists use absolute values, either in text or in tables, to express variations in study parameters. Some quantify effects by expressing the changes (increases or decreases) as compared with the appropriate control values. Others qualify the effects using severity modifiers such as minimal, marked, etc., with or without quantifying the changes. This communicates the author's interpretation of the changes, and requires her/his scientific expertise to reflect what has occurred biologically. Still others prefer to accentuate the changes seen by placing the control or pretest value in parentheses next to the effect described. Using this approach assumes that the reader has sufficient knowledge to make her/his own interpretation of the data, and additionally assumes that the interpretation will be the same as your own! When deciding which approach to use, remember your audience, and take into consideration its level of expertise in clinical pathology. If your reader is not knowledgeable in this area, you are strongly advised to qualify as well as quantify your results.

Using percentages to quantify changes is acceptable, but for changes greater than 100%, this terminology can become confusing. The interpretation of your prose can become the reader's exercise in semantics. Consider the case where the control mean value for alkaline phosphatase is 50 IU/liter and the high-dose value is 150 IU/liter. An increase reported as "+200% as compared with control values" may be interpreted in at least two ways:

1. 200% of the control value (200% × 50 mg/l), or 100 IU/l
2. 200% greater than the control value [(200% × 50 IU/l) + 50 IU/l], or 150 IU/l (the true high-dose value).

A reader may consider these or other options, and not know which one to choose. This may force him/her to go to tables in a separate section to look for the actual high-dose value, which means that you have not achieved the clarity of expression that you wish to be the hallmark of your report. The term "-fold" may be used as an alternative in this instance. If the above-mentioned change is reported as a threefold increase over the control value, the only conclusion that the reader can reach is that the high-dose value is triple the control value.

Some clinical pathologists will use a combination of terminologies to express data in a single report, e.g. using percentage change to describe some chemistry parameters, -fold change to describe enzyme or hematology changes, and absolute numbers to describe specific individual parameters. They make their choices based on experience in dealing with the types of numbers generated by these parameters (e.g. since doubling or tripling of serum sodium or chloride is biologically impossible, one would not use the term "-fold" to describe increases in these parameters). Others prefer to choose one method of quantification for all parameters. Still others do not quantify results at all in the text, but provide tables for this purpose. The options available to you will likely be dictated by your experience and your department's report-writing policy.

Remember that food consumption, body weight and other types of data in the report will require quantification as well, and that other authors may report their data differently. Thus, it may be advisable to standardize the terminology used for quantifying data among the departments contributing to the toxicology report so as not to confuse the reader. Again, this will depend on your laboratory's report-writing policy.

There may be compound-related changes which can be considered side-effects of clinical signs or histopathologic changes resulting from compound administration. These changes should be identified as such, along with the clinical sign(s) to which the effects are attributed. For example, severe diarrhea can lead to dehydration, which in turn can cause increased total red blood cell count, hemoglobin and hematocrit as well as increased total protein and urea nitrogen. Glucose levels could also increase on account of the stress experienced by the affected animals. None of these clinical pathology findings is directly attributable to administration of the compound, but they are all secondary to clinical signs caused by the compound. They should be described after primary compound-related effects are discussed.

Compound-related changes should not be confused with other "treatment-related" changes. These encompass changes resulting from the vehicle used, the method of administration of the product tested, and physiologic effects caused by study procedure (e.g. decreased red blood cell counts resulting from repeated bleedings). Treatment-related changes not directly attributed to the compound should be discussed later in the Results section.

7.2.2 *Are the Changes Dose-related? At What Dose Do They Appear?*

The strongest indicator of a compound-related effect is the presence of a dose-relationship. Stating that such a relationship exists accentuates the conclusion that an effect is compound-related. Intimately tied to this are the dose levels at which the effect is seen. Affected dose levels *MUST* be clearly stated, preferably using the numerical values of doses instead of terms like "high-dose" or "mid-dose".

7.2.3 What Is the Incidence of the Change?

The incidence of an effect reflects the number of animals with values outside the defined reference range for a given parameter. It is generally reported as a fraction, e.g. 2/4 or 9/10 animals affected. The incidence can often help to determine whether or not an effect is related to compound administration and, more specifically, at what dose level it begins to be manifested. For example, imagine that a change is clearly identified in the mean of the high-dose group of a study. If the mean value of the intermediate-dose group is slightly different from that of the control group, yet several individual animal values within the group are outside the range of individual control values, there is more evidence to suggest that animals at this dose level are affected by the compound.

Incidence is reported *only* when it provides important additional information. It can effectively be reported in text: "Compound-treated males had moderate to marked bilirubin scores [2/5 at 5 mg/kg (moderate), 1/5 at 10 mg/kg (marked), 1/5 at 20 mg/kg (marked)] which were not observed in the pretest urinalysis", as well as in tables (see Example 7.3).

Example 7.3 Tabular presentation of incidence

Table 7.1 PP 75167: 1-Month oral toxicity study in beagle dogs – compound-related clinical chemistry findings on day 28: percentage change[a] and incidence[b].

Parameter	Sex	Dose (mg/kg/day)			
		5	10	20	40
ALP[c]	M	—[e]	—	—	+285% (4/5)*
	F	—	—	+223% (1/3)*	+580% (2/4)*[f]
5'NUC[d]	M	—	—	—	+500% (5/5)*
	F	—	—	+150% (1/3)*	+300% (4/4)*[f]
Cholesterol	M	+48% (2/3)	+48% (2/3)	+67% (2/3)	+48% (4/5)*
	F	+40% (1/3)	+35% (2/3)	+31% (3/3)	+79% (3/4)*[f]

[a]Percentage change is expressed in relation to mean control values. [b]Number of animals with values outside the reference range. [c]Alkaline phosphatase. [d]5'-Nucleotidase. [e]Values were within reference range. [f]One female died on day 15 of the study. *$p < 0.05$.

Data from individual animals are not discussed unless they help to clarify a result. Consider the following scenario: In a study in which anemia and thrombocytopenia are expected compound-related changes, a dose-related effect is observed. The incidence is one out of four at the lowest dose affected, two out of four at the middle dose, and four out of four at the highest dose. The paragraph shown as Example 7.4 was placed in the Results section. The information justifies asserting that 0.1 mg/kg should be considered a no-effect dose.

Example 7.4   Use of data from an individual animal to clarify a result

One 0.1 mg/kg male (No. 2003) was sacrificed during the study (day 83) because of severe anemia and thrombocytopenia associated with increased prothrombin time, reduced fibrinogen and neutrophilic leukocytosis. These changes were compatible with disseminated intravascular coagulation, which was interpreted to be secondary to the presence of a permanent intravenous indwelling catheter (the route of compound administration), and a resulting bacterial septicemia (confirmed by light microscopy). This effect was not considered to be related to compound administration.

7.2.4   Is the Effect Noted in Both Sexes?

An effect does not need to be found in both sexes to be interpreted as a compound-related effect. The differences in metabolism and hormone status between sexes sometimes make one sex more susceptible or resistant to a given toxicologic effect. These differences are very important to note, particularly in relation to eventual clinical trials in the case of pharmaceutical compounds.

7.2.5   Is There a Progressive Increase in the Severity and/or Incidence of the Change?

In studies of several months' duration, the progression of the severity of effects is important to note. When necessary, the specific sampling periods at which effects are noted should be discussed. In large-animal studies, the number of animals having progressing signs (the incidence) is equally important to track and discuss in the Results section. Detailed results may be reported in a table (see Example 7.5).

Example 7.5   Tabular presentation of variation of incidence with time during a lengthy study

Table 7.2   PP 34163: 6-Month oral toxicity study in beagle dogs – incidence[a] of compound-related increases in blood urea nitrogen (BUN) and creatinine.

Parameter	BUN						Creatinine					
Sex	Male			Female			Male			Female		
Treatment day	D32	D93	D179	D32	D93	D179	D32	D93	D179	D32	D93	D179
Dose (mg/kg/day)												
10	—[b]	—	—	1/5	2/5	3/5	1/5	—	1/5	2/5	2/5	3/5
30	—	1/5	2/5	4/5	4/5	5/5	3/5	3/5	3/5	1/5	4/5	3/5

[a]Number of animals with values outside the reference range. [b]Values were within the reference range.

It is important to remember that certain clinical pathology parameters will spontaneously change over time (e.g. decreasing alkaline phosphatase levels in young dogs), and that these should not be interpreted as effects related to compound administration. Indeed, knowledge of these normal biological shifts in parameters will increase your ability to identify changes which *should* be attributed to the compound, such as stable or increasing alkaline phosphatase levels in treated groups while control group levels decrease as would be expected.

7.2.6 Is the Effect Reversible? Is the Recovery Partial or Complete? How Is It Manifested?

In studies in which there are multiple sampling periods, changes noted on one sampling date may not appear on subsequent sampling dates. In this instance, one should carefully consider whether or not the change is transient but compound-related, or whether it may be considered unrelated to compound administration. Certain sporadic and transient changes merit discussion because they may be important markers for clinical trials (e.g. transient increases in liver enzyme values, decreases in red blood cell parameters or platelets). Thus, even a change in one animal may be compound-related (see Example 7.6). Prior knowledge of how the compound, or compounds of its class, is expected to behave can greatly help determine the significance of such effects.

Example 7.6   Discussion of transient change

> The creatinine in male dog No.15 (50 mg/kg/day) increased twofold from day 3 (8 mg/l) to day 14 (16 mg/l), then decreased to reference range by day 28 (9 mg/l). Though transient, this increase exceeded the concurrent study control range and reference range values for dogs of this age and sex, and was considered to be compound-related. Associated histopathologic changes were observed in the kidneys. All other values were comparable between treated and control groups and did not vary significantly during the course of the study.

In studies in which there is a reversibility or recovery period, animals in which changes were noted at the end of the treatment phase may be examined at the end of an additional period during which treatment is withheld. Here, one looks for a trend toward regression of the effects noted during the treatment period. For more severe changes, the reversal may not be complete, because of the generally short duration of the reversibility period as compared with the treatment period; but milder changes may return completely to reference range values.

Compound-induced effects sometimes cause additional changes in related clinical pathology parameters; these secondary changes may indicate a biological response to the compound-induced effect. For example, decreased total red blood cells, hemoglobin, and hematocrit (primary changes) noted during the treatment period may increase by the end of the reversibility period, with an increase in reticulocytes (secondary change) providing additional evidence of recovery. A distinction between these two types of effect should be made in the text when possible.

Finally, data gathered at the end of the reversibility period may be used to confirm or reject the hypothesis that questionable variations in clinical pathology analytes observed during the treatment period are actually caused by compound administration. Consider a case where mild elevations in liver enzymes are consistently found in two out of five high-dose monkeys during the 28-day treatment period, and yet there are no increases in the high-dose mean when compared with mean control values. Could these individual variations be due to a direct effect of the compound administered? If the enzyme levels in these two animals are found to be within reference range at the end of the reversibility period, one can say with more confidence that the elevations observed during treatment were compound-related. Again, prior knowledge of the expected effect of the compound can help make this determination.

7.3 Putting Findings into Perspective

Depending on the style of report writing used in your company, you may discuss the relevance of each group of findings in the same section in which you present the results, or in a separate section altogether. Whatever the style used, the data should be put into proper perspective and, when possible or appropriate, the following issues regarding compound-related effects should be addressed.

1   Indicate whether compound-related findings are due to a direct effect of the compound, or are considered to be secondary changes.

2   If there is an attempt to establish a no-effect dose, or to convince the reader that compound-related effects present at the lowest dose are not toxicologically relevant, the potential significance of these effects must be clarified (e.g. severity, incidence, relation to reference range values).

3   Make any possible correlations with in-life observations, anatomic pathologic findings and other data.

4   When possible, address whether or not the effect is expected with the class of compound. If so, briefly describe the mechanism (if known). Is it an exaggerated pharmacological effect? Here, references to earlier studies with the same compound, compounds with the same pharmacological activity, or scientific literature clarifying the meaning of the effect may be used: for example, "Increased cholesterol was previously observed in a 14-day toxicity study in rats receiving 20 mg/kg PP 23369, but to a lesser extent. Increases in calcium, albumin and total protein associated with changes in hematology indicate hemoconcentration which is probably secondary to the known diuretic action of this compound (Author, year)". Use of references, whether they be to studies done in your facility, in contract labs, or to scientific literature, should be harmonized throughout the report. It is strongly recommended that the actual text of the reference be kept short (as in the example above), and to have a full reference list at the end of the report.

5   The biological/toxicological significance (or lack thereof) of the effect should be discussed: for example, "The minimal effect on PT and aPTT observed after

treatment with 15 mg/kg/day of PP 11506 was not considered to be biologically significant, because all values noted in compound-treated animals were near or within the range of values found in control animals".

6 Discuss whether or not the effect in the test species is relevant to man. Certain species have particular ways of reacting to the administration of xenobiotics which have little or uncertain relevance in humans. For example, certain regulatory agencies may require the evaluation of creatine phosphokinase (CPK) and lactic dehydrogenase (LDH) as part of the biochemistry panel for toxicity studies. The reference ranges for CPK and LDH are very wide in normal animals, and levels are susceptible to variations resulting from animal handling and sample collection. Increases in these enzymes can be of questionable significance in animals, and are not likely to be predictive of toxic effects in humans.

Once all compound-related effects have been addressed, additional treatment-related effects should be described. This section of the report should be brief. If the report-writing policy at your company separates results from discussion, and if the observed changes are not considered to be important, then describe these effects in the Results section. However, if treatment-related changes are important in the overall interpretation of study results, then they should be placed in the Discussion section. Examples 7.7 to 7.9 show some ways of dealing with this subject.

Example 7.7   Vehicle-related effects

Variations in other clinical pathology parameters (urine volume and urine osmolarity) were not considered to be related to treatment with PP 27567 since they were also observed in the vehicle-treated control group.

Example 7.8   Pathological effects secondary to the route of compound administration

Increases in RBC and WBC parameters and reductions in total protein, albumin, globulin and A/G ratios in treated and control animals were attributed to inflammation at injection sites.

Example 7.9   Physiological effects secondary to study procedure

Minimal reductions in RBC count (−2% to −6%, in males and −7% to −11%, in females) in rats at all dose levels, including controls, were interpreted to be the result of reduced blood volume following blood collection at 2-day intervals. Because the compound caused a primary decrease in total RBCs, this methodology-induced decrease interfered with the assessment of the severity of the compound's effect on red cell counts at all dose levels.

At the end of the Results section, variations which are not considered to be treatment-related should be addressed as simply and as succinctly as possible. An example of a short but all-encompassing paragraph which could be useful is the following: "Other variations were observed among groups and at different sampling periods. While some of these variations reached statistical significance, they were near or within the limits of our reference range values (control values and/or pretest values and/or historical data), and no consistent trends were observed that could be attributed to treatment".

In Conclusion

The Clinical Pathology section of the toxicology report should be written simply, clearly and with the reader's needs in mind. It should contain the fewest words possible to explain your ideas, without sacrificing comprehensibility and clarity. Lead your reader so that, with minimal effort, she/he can understand and accept your conclusions with regard to data interpretation.

8

Anatomic Pathology

T. HODGE

Rhône-Poulenc Rorer, Drug Safety Department, Vitry sur Seine, France

and S. GOSSELIN

ITR Laboratories Canada Inc., Montreal, Canada

The Anatomic Pathology section of a regulatory toxicology report contains information related to organ weight changes, necropsy findings and histopathologic evaluation. Depending on the objectives of the study (single-dose study, reproductive study, range-finding study, investigative study, etc.), some or all of these parameters may be excluded. Depending on your laboratory or company report-writing policy, the Anatomic Pathology section is either an integral part of the regulatory toxicology report or a separate report written as an annex and included as an appendix of the regulatory toxicology report. It may consist either of results with a discussion within each respective subsection (organ weight, necropsy, histopathology) of the narrative, or only the results – with an overall discussion of all results placed at the end of the toxicology report. The writing philosophy of this Guide is based on clarity of data presentation and interpretation, flow of ideas and a coherence of the logical relation between information from different sources; therefore, only examples of an Anatomic Pathology section which would immediately follow the Clinical Pathology section are presented here.

In the Materials and Methods, in addition to the standard list of tissues to be examined, the dose levels, organs evaluated during the treatment and recovery (if applicable) periods and the special techniques used (histochemistry, electron microscopy, immunocytochemistry, morphometry, etc.) should be mentioned. A statement on peer review may be included.

In general, the order of presentation in the Results should begin with organ weights, followed by necropsy, then by histopathology. Identify as clearly as possible which effects are compound-induced and which ones are secondary to the vehicle or the technical procedure. Avoid detailed description of spontaneous or spurious events which may unnecessarily confuse the reader. Naturally occurring effects should be mentioned if they interfere with the evaluation of compound-related findings or if the administration of the compound exacerbates an effect/lesion of a spontaneous nature. If the discussion of the results follows each subsection, detailed significance of the associated results (correlations with in-life observations, clinical pathology findings, organ weight changes, etc.) are included in the most appropriate subsection, and only referred to in the remaining subsections.

8.1 Organ Weights

Organ weight changes are the differences, expressed in percentages, between treated and non-treated groups in terms of relative and absolute organ weights. Since body weight changes have already been addressed in the section on in-life measurements, these should be mentioned only in terms of explaining changes in organ weights. If body weight changes are substantial, it may be preferable to express the relative organ weight values with respect to brain weight rather than to body weight. Because of the wider variability between individual body weights in large animals compared with small animals, relative organ weights are more useful than absolute organ weights in these species. Therefore, if a table within the text is appropriate in large-animal studies, only the relative organ weights should be tabulated. A text table should be used when multiple or complex organ weight changes are present. The organ weights of animals found dead during the course of a study should be taken, since they may provide useful information on reasons for early deaths; but may be excluded from the final calculation of means.

The narrative should begin by describing compound-related changes. If there are no compound-related effects, simply state that no compound-related effects were observed in the organ weights. If compound-related effects are present (whether the changes are statistically significant or not), this should be stated in the first sentence (Example 8.1). Subsequently, the organ weight changes should be qualified in terms of whether the absolute weights, the relative weights, or both are altered; these changes should be expressed as a mean percentage change (increase or decrease) compared with the appropriate control mean values (usually the vehicle-control values). In addition, the following points, if applicable, should be mentioned.

- Is the change dose-related? If so, at what dose does it begin? Often, a slight change in organ weights which is not statistically significant and would not otherwise be worthy of mention, may indicate the beginning of a trend if the organ weights at higher doses indicate a clear compound effect.

- Is the change statistically significant? Often when there is a dose-response related to an organ weight change, the changes observed at the lower dose/doses may not be statistically significant. Therefore, do not rely on statistical significance to indicate a compound effect.

- Is it noted in both or only in one sex? If an organ weight change is present in only one sex, try to relate the change to other parameters measured in the study, i.e. clinical pathology changes or the presence or absence of histo-pathological findings, which can substantiate whether or not the change is compound-related.

- What is the incidence at each dose/sex affected? It is usually not included as part of the report; however, it may help in interpreting the significance of the results and establish a dose-relationship. If there is more than one organ affected and if changes are complex, a text table may be appropriate.

Example 8.1

> Compound-related organ weight changes were noted for the liver in males
> at 10 mg/kg/day and in both sexes at 25 mg/kg/day and for the testis at
> 25 mg/kg/day.
>
> When compared with the mean vehicle-control values, statistically significant
> dose-related increases in mean absolute and relative liver weights were noted
> in males treated at 10 and 25 mg/kg/day (+20 and +40%, respectively). In females,
> a similar increase in liver weight (+30%) was limited to the 25 mg/kg/day group.
> In addition, the 25 mg/kg/day males had lower (−25%) mean absolute and relative
> testis weights. Liver and testicular changes correlated microscopically with
> hepatocellular hypertrophy and bilateral degeneration of the seminiferous
> tubules, respectively (see Histopathology). There were no other organ weight
> changes which were considered related to treatment with compound PP 27567.
> Several other differences in group mean absolute and/or relative organ weights
> between control and treated groups achieved statistical significance, but these
> were considered incidental and not compound-related as they were slight, not
> dose-related, observed in only one sex and/or unaccompanied by correlated
> morphologic findings.

- Are organ weight changes mainly due to changes in body weight?
- If a recovery group is used, is the recovery partial or complete?
- Values that are clearly out of the range of the control values or statistically
  flagged, but not considered compound-related and/or of pathologic significance, should be addressed in one to two sentences with appropriate
  qualifications as to their significance. State the reason for these differences if
  known, or supply a statement similar to the following: "Some differences in
  organ weights were observed among individuals but were considered incidental
  since they were sporadic, unaccompanied by morphologic findings, and/or
  without relation to dose or sex". The organ weight changes may be specifically
  cited if they are few in number and if the citation clarifies the reader's
  perspective.
- The number of animals per group, normal population variation, tissue
  trimming techniques and degree of exsanguination at necropsy may have an
  effect on organ weights and should be addressed in the narrative if they are
  considered to have affected the evaluation.

In the last paragraph of the organ weight section (RDRD structure) or in the
overall discussion (modified IMRAD structure), the data should be put into
perspective and, when possible, the following questions should be addressed.

- Are there any correlations with clinical observations, clinical pathology, gross
  or microscopic findings, etc.? These should be mentioned with reference to
  the respective section.
- Is there a no-effect level? If there is an attempt to establish a no-effect dose
  level while dose-related findings are described at the lowest dose level, the
  toxicological significance of the finding at that level should be clarified (minimal

incidence and/or severity, within normal historical range, etc.) (Example 8.3).

- Is the change a consequence of the known pharmacological activity of the compound? For example, a compound with enzyme-inducing activity might be expected to cause increased liver weights (Example 8.2).

Example 8.2

Table 8.1 PP 27567: 6-Month oral toxicity in rats – compound-related changes in mean relative organ weights.[a]

Organ	Males			Females		
	50 mg/kg	100 mg/kg	200 mg/kg	50 mg/kg	100 mg/kg	200 mg/kg
Liver						
%change	+12*	+15*	+36*	+16	+22*	+42*
incidence	4/10	7/10	9/10	6/10	8/9	10/10
Adrenals						
% change	+37	+25	+19	+10	+7	+5
incidence	3/10	3/10	4/10	2/10	1/9	2/10
Heart						
% change	–	+8	+20	–	–	–
incidence	–	–	2/10	–	–	–

*$p < 0.05$
[a]Mean compound-treated group values compared with mean vehicle-control values

The administration of PP 27567 was associated with:

- dose-related increases (incidence and severity) in mean relative liver weight at 50, 100 and 200 mg/kg/day in both sexes. This effect correlated with dose-related increases in mean absolute liver weight in males (+15% to +35% of mean control values) and in females (+16% to + 42% of mean control values)
- increases in mean absolute and relative adrenal weight at 50, 100 and 200 mg/kg/day in males only
- increases in mean absolute and relative heart weights at 100 and 200 mg/kg/day in males only.

At all dose levels, higher liver weight correlated with hepatocellular hyper-trophy, while adrenal changes correlated with diffuse hypertrophy of the zona fasciculata of the adrenal cortex. Individual heart weight increases were within the range of values observed in controls and were therefore considered to have little toxicological significance. Increased heart weight may be secondary to the tachycardia observed at these dose levels which is a known pharmacologic effect of the compound (see Cardiovascular parameters in the Clinical Observation section) (Author, year).

Example 8.3

Table 8.2 Mean absolute liver weight increases in female rats receiving PP 27567 for 6 months.[a]

Dose (mg/kg/day)	5	20	80
% change	+8	+22*	+32**
incidence	2/10	5/10	10/10

*$p<0.05$; ** $p<0.01$
[a]Mean compound-treated group values compared with mean vehicle-control values
Note: a similar weight increase was observed with mean relative liver weights

There were no microscopic findings associated with the liver weight changes. Minimal increases in liver weight at 5 mg/kg/day noted in only 2/10 females were considered to have little, if any, toxicological significance.

8.2 Necropsy

Observations at necropsy should be used primarily to identify the extent of the compound-related lesions and any other lesions which are better described grossly, such as skin lesions, injections site lesions, etc. (Examples 8.4 to 8.7). If there are no compound-related findings, simply state that no compound-related findings were observed at necropsy. If compound-related findings are present, indicate the number of animals affected per sex and per group for each finding. Note whether the gross findings correlate with clinical observations or microscopic findings. Summarize all non-compound-related gross findings in one succinct sentence or

Example 8.4

Skin lesions at injection sites (thickening/swelling, erosions/ulcers, exudation, dark firm, edema) were observed in all compound-treated groups and reflect the irritant nature of the compound when administered subcutaneously.

Example 8.5

Compound-related gross findings were noted only in the testis and thymus of the 10 mg/kg/day animals. Small testes and thymuses were observed in 10/10 males. These lesions correlated with microscopic findings of testicular degeneration and lymphoid depletion of the thymus (see Histopathology). Following the recovery period, small testes were still present in 4/5 males while compound-related changes in the thymus were no longer present. All other gross observations were incidental and spontaneous in nature and bore no relation to treatment with PP 27567.

---

paragraph. Refrain from going deeply into details, since the final diagnoses will be confirmed by light microscopy.

Following the description of any morphologic findings, a paragraph on mortality and any associated gross findings should follow (Examples 8.8 to 8.11). Depending on the philosophy of the company, this section could be part of Clinical Observations and the result of a team-effort between Toxicology and Pathology. If there was no mortality in the study, state that all animals survived until the end of the study. If animals were sacrificed early or found dead during the study, state whether or not these deaths were compound-related. Early deaths that are related to gavage accidents can be mentioned here along with any histopathological findings confirming the diagnosis of a gavage accident. These animals need not be referred to again. If there were multiple deaths, describe the number of dead animals per group and comment on the cause of death.

Example 8.6

Compound-related gross findings were characterized by:

- thin body at 200 mg/kg (2/5 males, 1/5 females)
- edematous pericardial and thymic fat at 200 mg/kg/day (2/5 males, 1/5 females)
- small thymus at 200 mg/kg/day (4/5 males, 3/5 females)
- enlarged spleen at 200 (3/5 males) and 100 mg/kg/day (1/5 males)

These findings were attributed to anemia and weight loss (see Clinical Observations and Clinical Pathology).

Example 8.7

Compound-related gross findings were noted in the liver and testis. Enlargement of the liver was observed in 13/20 males and in 9/20 females treated at 25 mg/kg/day. Small, soft testes were noted in 14/20 males treated at 25 mg/kg/day. Gross observations in the liver and testis correlated with the microscopic observations described in the Histopathology section. All other gross observations were incidental findings typical of those routinely observed in Sprague-Dawley rats of this age.

Example 8.8

Four animals (2/10 females at 50 mg/kg/day, 1/10 males at 100 mg/kg/day and 1/10 females at 200 mg/kg/day) did not survive until the scheduled necropsy. The two 50 mg/kg/day females (No. 91: found dead; No. 100: sacrificed as moribund) had gross observations compatible with gavage error (see Table X). The cause of poor condition requiring sacrifice for the remaining animals was undetermined from gross or microscopic examination.

Example 8.9

One of the females (No. 38) at 200 mg/kg/day died on day 8 of the study because of extensive hemorrhage into the gastric and intestinal lumen. The gastrointestinal hemorrhages were the result of gastric mucosal ulcers, probably secondary to severe repeated emesis and retching (Author, year). Emesis has been previously reported in association with the oral administration of high doses of this compound, where death was often preceded by sodium and chloride imbalance (references).

Example 8.10

The only unscheduled death occurred in a 10 mg/kg/day male (No. 034) on day 27. Necropsy observations on the kidney, lung, liver and spleen corresponded microscopically with acute tubular necrosis, pulmonary edema and congestion with hemorrhages in the liver and spleen. While these changes probably contributed to the animal's death, their cause could not be determined. However, the changes are not considered to be related to compound, because of their isolated occurrence and the absence of a dose relationship.

Example 8.11

Gross pathologic findings observed in moribund animals were the following:

- red-brown staining of the fur around the nose in rats receiving 500 and 1000 mg/kg/day
- yellow-green or red-brown staining of the fur of the abdomen in animals given 500 (females) and 1000 mg/kg/day (both sexes)
- erosion(s)/ulcer(s) of the stomach in animals given 500 and 1000 mg/kg/day (both sexes)
- decreased size of the thymus in animals given 500 and 1000 mg/kg/day (both sexes).

The lesions in the stomach were confirmed microscopically to be erosions. The decreased size of the thymus was consistent with a decreased thymus weight and lymphoid depletion observed microscopically. These non-specific findings are frequently noted in rats in poor condition.

8.3 Histopathology

The major responsibility of the toxicologic pathologist is to identify and describe microscopic changes induced by a test article in the tissues of laboratory animals. These changes need to be correlated with clinical observations, alterations in clinical pathology parameters and organ weights, and their significance must be interpreted taking into account their relationship with the amount of compound to which the animals have been exposed. The data should be put into proper perspective for a reader who may have limited training or experience in toxicologic pathology. Therefore, the histopathology results must be written clearly, succinctly, accurately and be presented logically.

At the time of this writing, the Society of Toxicologic Pathologists in the USA and the Registry of Industrial Toxicology Animal-data (RITA) in Germany are undertaking the formidable task of standardizing the vocabulary used in toxicologic pathology. Historically, the language of pathology has been complex, confusing, sometimes ambiguous and often subjective. With pathologists themselves often in disagreement over terminology, it is not surprising that readers who are not pathologists are often confused when presented with pages of text filled with unfamiliar and sometimes "frightening" terms. The reader, who may be a biologist or a pharmacologist in a regulatory agency, is often left to his own devices to put pathologic changes into perspective relative to human risk assessment.

A well-defined glossary of diagnoses should be decided upon within an organization in order to impose uniformity among pathologists. In addition to ensuring that all pathologists in an organization use the same terminology to describe the same histopathologic finding, a glossary is important both in the production of uniform reports and for establishing historical databases within an organization. The number of diagnoses should not be exhaustive, but rather, an effort should be made to combine or "lump" similar pathologic processes together. This is especially important for long-term studies where there are large numbers of findings. Also, since the difference between hyperplasia and neoplasia of a particular cell type is often vague, it is important to make a distinction between the two. When a hyperplastic or neoplastic lesion is considered a test article effect in a carcinogenicity study, it is desirable both to combine and separate the possible stages of that lesion (hyperplasia, benign and malignant neoplasia) for statistical purposes. To make these manipulations, strict definitions regarding the morphologic boundaries between malignant and benign neoplasia and hyperplasia need to be specified.

Standardization and definition also should be given to descriptive terminology, such as severity degrees (e.g., minimal, mild, moderate and marked) and distribution modifiers (e.g., focal, multifocal, locally extensive, diffuse, unilateral and bilateral). This is of paramount importance in decreasing diagnostic subjectivity, in putting the severity of findings into perspective regarding their overall toxicologic importance, and ultimately in arriving at the best decisions related to risk assessment.

The histopathology section should begin by stating that Compound X either did or did not produce an effect. If it did, state the change, organ, sex, and dose groups affected. If numerous changes are present, list the target organs and describe the changes in subsequent sentences/paragraphs. Text tables may be used when there are multiple findings. The text should concentrate on the concise presentation of compound-related findings, and long, detailed histopathologic descriptions should be avoided.

In the first sentence/paragraph, identify the dose levels which are affected along with the target organ, the number of animals per dose group and per sex, and its associated change (Examples 8.12 and 8.13). If possible, list the organs in order

Example 8.12

Compound-related histopathologic findings were noted at the end of the treatment period in multiple organs in animals treated at 1 and 5 mg/kg/day. These findings consisted of hypocellularity of the bone marrow at 1 and 5 mg/kg, focal or multifocal atrophy of the seminiferous tubules of the testes with individual spermatocyte necrosis at 5 mg/kg, and single cell necrosis and increased numbers of mitotic figures in salivary and lacrimal glands at 1 and 5 mg/kg. All were considered to be related to the anti-mitotic properties of this compound. After a 4-week recovery period, treatment-related findings persisted only in the testis, epididymides and lacrimal glands.

of importance: e.g. liver would be listed before harderian gland. If the study includes a recovery period, mention whether or not the recovery occurs and, if so, whether it is partial or complete (Example 8.12).

After the compound-related changes have been listed, a description of the changes, organ by organ, should follow. Diagnostic terms should be defined keeping in mind that most readers of the report will not be pathologists. During the description of the lesions, one or two sentences can be used to describe their distribution and severity. Distribution modifiers (focal, multifocal, diffuse, locally extensive) and severity modifiers (minimal, mild, moderate, marked, severe) are useful to put findings into perspective. Histopathologic lesions may be compound-related because of their distribution or their severity, even if the incidence of the finding is not increased. In other words, a dose response related to severity or distribution must be considered as well as a dose response related to incidence. If a special technique such as histochemistry or electron microscopy helped confirm or supplement the initial histopathological diagnoses, it should be mentioned.

For each histopathologic finding, briefly mention any possible correlation or association with organ weight changes, gross findings and ante-mortem findings (Clinical Observations, Clinical Pathology, Toxicokinetic, etc.).

If possible, explain findings based on the known pharmacological properties of the compound. Instead of being part of the Results, this could be included in the Discussion, depending on the philosophy of the organization. This can help to put into perspective and often minimize the importance of certain findings. Explain if the finding is expected with this class of compounds or is secondary to an exaggerated pharmacological effect (Example 8.13).

Lesions related to route of administration, methodology, or secondary to the vehicle should be grouped together and be kept to a minimum of one or two sentences. Inflammatory lesions related to irritant compounds given subcutaneously or intravenously or ocular lesions related to orbital sinus bleeding are examples of this type of finding.

In some instances, certain histopathologic findings may have no or little relevance to man, e.g. thyroid follicular cell hypertrophy/hyperplasia in rats secondary to microsomal enzyme induction. Findings may also be limited to one species. Any known information related to species specificity will help to minimize and put into perspective a compound-related effect. Interpretation of such changes in this manner should be accompanied by references.

Finally, group all non-compound-related findings into one sentence or one succinct paragraph. State why these changes are not considered compound-related (similar incidence in controls, common findings in this strain, incidental, spontaneous, developmental, caused by animal handling, etc. – Example 8.14). If spontaneous lesions interfere with the proper evaluation of possible compound-induced lesions, this should be mentioned (Example 8.15).

Example 8.13

Compound-related histopathologic findings were noted in the liver and thyroid at 25 mg/kg/day, and in the testis at 10 and 25 mg/kg/day. In the liver, centrilobular hepatocellular hypertrophy was observed in 10/20 males and in 7/20 females treated at 25 mg/kg/day, and was characterized by increased size and cytoplasmic eosinophilia of centrilobular hepatocytes. Severity ranged from mild to moderate in affected males and from minimal to mild in affected females and correlated with the increased liver weight observed in these groups. Centrilobular hepatocellular hypertrophy is most likely the result of increased hepatic microsomal enzyme activity induced by PP 27567, as demonstrated in a previous study (Reference).

In the thyroid, multifocal to diffuse hyperplasia was noted in 8/20 males and in 5/20 females treated at 25 mg/kg/day. It was characterized by small follicles which were lined by columnar epithelial cells with finely vacuolated cytoplasm surrounding retracted, basophilic colloid. This change was frequently associated with centrilobular hepatocellular hypertrophy, and could be related to altered hepatic clearance of thyroid hormones resulting from increased hepatic microsomal enzyme activity induced by PP 27567 (Reference).

Finally, in the testis, degeneration of the seminiferous tubules was observed in 13/20 males treated at 25 mg/kg/day and in 7/20 males treated at 10 mg/kg/day, and was characterized by degeneration of spermatocytes in some tubules, associated with a clear loss of germ cells and retention of Sertoli cells in others. Severity and distribution of this change were dose-related (minimal to focal at 10 mg/kg/day and mild to multifocal at 25 mg/kg/day) and correlated with decreased testicular weights and with the gross necropsy observation of small, soft testes at 25 mg/kg/day.

All other microscopic findings were incidental and spontaneous in nature and were not attributed to the compound.

Example 8.14

There were no compound-related findings in this study. All microscopic findings were either related to orbital sinus bleeding, to venipuncture, or were incidental and of the type routinely observed in Sprague-Dawley rats of this age.

Example 8.15

The administration of PP 27567 was associated with histopathological findings which consisted of moderate to marked tubular dilatation, basophilia and degeneration in the kidneys at doses of 50 and 250 mg/kg/day (4/6 and 10/10 animals, respectively). At 10 mg/kg/day (2/6 animals), the findings were limited to minimal to mild renal tubular changes. Spontaneous renal lesions (interstitial inflammation) were noted in several animals, including controls; these spontaneous lesions interfered with the interpretation of the renal findings, particularly in the 10 mg/kg/day group.

8.4 Reporting the Results of Carcinogenicity Studies

When reporting the results of a carcinogenicity study the writer must keep in mind that the primary purpose of the study is to identify compound-related neoplastic and/or hyperplastic changes. If non-neoplastic changes have occurred during the course of a carcinogenicity study, it is possible that these lesions have been identified previously in studies of shorter duration. In this case, they should be discussed briefly after the section(s) on neoplastic and hyperplastic findings, and appropriate references given. Along these lines, it is not unusual to observe exaggerated pharmacological effects of compounds after prolonged administration, and this should also be discussed briefly if observed.

Carcinogenicity studies may or may not have clinical pathology or organ weight data to analyze as part of the results. If these sections are present, however, they should be dealt with as outlined previously. Often the only clinical pathology parameters examined are those related to hematology, especially if the compound is suspected to have either a suppressive or stimulatory effect on any of the blood cell lines.

Cause of death is often dealt with in the histopathology section of a carcinogenicity report (Example 8.16). State what the major causes of death were in the preterminal animals, e.g. pituitary adenoma or spontaneous renal disease in rats, and express the incidence as a percentage value between groups. State whether or not the number of animals dying of undetermined causes was comparable between groups.

The histopathology section should begin by saying "up front" whether or not compound-related neoplastic or hyperplastic changes were observed (Example 8.17). If neoplastic changes were observed, the neoplasm and its associated organ should be listed in the first paragraph. Subsequently, try to devote a short but complete paragraph to describing and explaining each neoplastic change, its statistical significance, and the incidence of the change when coupled with any associated hyperplastic changes in a given organ. A neoplastic change in any given organ should be discussed in terms of the following possible combinations of reporting:

1   the total number of malignant tumors per sex per group
2   the total number of benign tumors per sex per group
3   the total combined number of benign and malignant tumors

4   the total number of proliferative lesions, i.e. malignant tumors + benign tumors + associated hyperplastic lesions.

The significance or cause of a given neoplastic or hyperplastic change can be discussed either in the histopathology Results or in an overall Discussion section depending on the philosophy of the organization.

Other topics which should be mentioned in the Results section include the following:

- whether or not the compound increased the total number of primary tumors
- if the compound affected the total number of clinically palpable or observable masses and the correlation of palpable masses with the histopathologic findings
- the number of systemic tumors, i.e. lymphomas, histiocytic sarcomas
- the total number of malignant tumors
- the tumor frequency in individual organs
- whether or not the compound influenced the time of onset of any tumors.

Example 8.16

The number of animals which died on the study or were euthanatized early in a moribund condition was comparable between the control and the treated groups. A total of 217 (72.3%) males and 187 (62.3%) females died or were euthanatized in a moribund condition during the 104-week treatment period. The individual group percentages for animals which died or were euthanatized early in a moribund condition were 65, 76.7, 75, 73.3 and 71.7% for males and 55, 63.3, 56.8, 66.7 and 70% for females for control groups 1 + 2 and the 5, 15 and 45 mg/kg/day groups, respectively. The major causes of death or moribundity among the preterminal animals were related to conditions frequently observed in Sprague-Dawley rats and included pituitary adenoma (the most frequent cause of death or moribundity among all groups), glomerulonephropathy, and mammary carcinoma in females. In addition, the number of animals dying of undetermined cause was comparably distributed among all groups, including controls.

Example 8.17

Treatment with PP27567 was associated with a slight but statistically significant ($p = 0.043$) increase in pheochromocytoma (a benign tumor of adrenal origin frequently observed in this strain of rats) in females treated with 45 mg/kg/day. The incidence of pheochromocytoma in this group (10.3%), although only slightly increased over that of the controls (2.5%) and slightly greater than that reported in most references for Sprague-Dawley rats (Authors, year), was considered a compound-related effect because similar effects have been observed with structurally related compounds (References).

Since the distinction between medullary hyperplasia and pheochromocytoma

continued

is often unclear and since the two diagnoses are most likely part of a continuum of the same lesion, the numerical values for these two findings were merged to provide a value for total proliferative medullary lesions. This combined value was also greater in the 45 mg/kg/day females than in the control females. The incidence of total proliferative medullary lesions in treated males was comparable to that of the control groups. In addition, there was no increase in bilateral tumors or in the incidence of animals which had both a pheochromocytoma and focal medullary hyperplasia. Focal medullary hyperplasia was composed of multifocal clusters of small, medullary cells which were darker and had larger nuclei than surrounding medullary cells. Focal medullary hyperplasia generally did not exhibit compression of the adjacent adrenal cortex. Pheochromocytomas were morphologically similar between all treatment groups, but their size ranged from masses only slightly larger than focal medullary hyperplasia with some compression of the adjacent medulla and cortex to large masses compressing the cortex into a thin rim of cells visible often only at one pole of the tumor. Vascular dilatation, congestion and hemorrhage were occasionally observed in tumors of all sizes.

Although most pheochromocytomas occurring in the 45 mg/kg/day females were found in animals that died or were euthanatized in a moribund condition, none was thought to be a cause of death or reason for early sacrifice. None of the pheochromocytomas displayed any evidence of malignancy and none of the animals bearing a pheochromocytoma had multiple endocrine neoplasia, except with pituitary adenoma, which was present in 93% of the female rats in this study and was present in similar numbers among all groups, including the controls.

The occurrences of two other neoplasms (hepatocellular adenoma in males and females, and testicular interstitial cell adenoma in males) were also statistically significant, but were clearly without relation to treatment with PP 27567 and were considered incidental findings. In males, the occurrence of hepatocellular adenoma was significant only by the trend analysis ($p = 0.048$) and represented only a slight increase in an extremely common tumor in this strain of rat. In females, the incidence of hepatocellular adenoma was significant ($p \leqslant 0.05$, Fisher's exact test) only in the 5 mg/kg/day animals and was not accompanied by a dose-response in the 15 and 45 mg/kg/day groups. Testicular interstitial cell adenoma was significant by the Fisher's exact test ($p \leqslant 0.05$) only in the 15 mg/kg/day males and was considered a fortuitous increase in the incidence of an infrequently occurring tumor. There were no occurrences of this tumor in the 45 mg/kg/day males.

There were no other increases in the incidence of other neoplastic or non-neoplastic findings which were considered to have a relationship to treatment with PP 27567. The total number of primary neoplasms (benign, malignant, or combined) and the total number of animals bearing a primary neoplasm among the compound-treated groups were comparable to the two control groups (Groups 1 and 2). In addition, PP 27567 had no effect on the number of clinically palpable masses, the tumor frequency in individual organs or the time of onset of any tumor.

continued

All other histopathologic findings in this study were spontaneous or incidental and were typical of those encountered in control male and female Sprague-Dawley rats used in long-term studies (Authors, year). These findings were observed with comparable frequency in both the control and compound-treated groups and none of these lesions was considered to have a relationship with the administration of PP 27567.

9

Developmental and Reproductive Toxicology

R. L. CLARK

Rhône-Poulenc Rorer Research and Development, Collegeville, USA

and G. COPPING

Rhône-Poulenc Rorer, Vitry sur Seine, France

9.1 Introduction

The principles and guidelines for writing toxicology study reports described in this book also apply to reports for developmental and reproductive toxicology studies. As is true for other reports, a developmental or reproductive toxicology report should be written to make it as easy as possible for the reader to understand the study design, results and interpretations. The author should keep in mind that the report will generally not be read cover to cover, but instead the reader will refer to the report to answer specific questions. This is why each section of the report should be as distinct and complete as possible. It should be recognized that, in most scientific writing, authors should express their point of view. The report should reflect the fact that the writer has carefully considered all the data and other information about the test compound and related test compounds and has arrived at an interpretation. The author's job is to convince the reader of that interpretation.

9.2 Terminology and Definitions

Some information concerning the development and use of the test species is prerequisite to understanding the terminology employed in developmental and reproductive toxicity studies. In this section we discuss the terminology used in reproduction toxicology reports. Terminology is summarized in Table 9.1.

9.2.1 Cohabitation and Mating

Pregnant rodents are usually obtained by cohabiting males and females at least overnight and often continuously until evidence of mating is observed. Rodents typically mate in the evening, and ovulation and fertilization occur in the morning following mating. Finding sperm or a seminal plug in the vagina in the morning is considered conclusive evidence of mating but a seminal plug in the cage tray may or may not be considered evidence of mating. The day that evidence of mating is found is variably considered to be either day 0 or day 1 of gestation (this chapter will consider this day to be day 0). Whether female rabbits are naturally mated during a brief cohabitation with a male or artificially inseminated, almost all laboratories consider the day of occurrence to be day 0 of gestation.

9.2.2 Embryonic Development

The period of development of the embryo (embryogenesis) begins with fertilization and is typically considered to conclude with the closure of the secondary (hard) palate (mouse – day 15; rat – day 16 to 17; rabbit – day 19) after which the conceptus is referred to as a fetus. Embryogenesis includes the period of major organogenesis which is considered to begin at implantation (approximately gestational day 5 to 6 in rodents and rabbits). When not wishing to specify either embryo or fetus, the term "conceptus" can be used or, as the adjective, "embryofetal". After delivery (caesarean section or birth), the rodent fetus is referred to as a pup.

9.2.3 Effects on the Conceptus

There are various types of effects on the conceptus (developmental toxicity). Treatment with the test compound may cause the death of the conceptus (resorption), effects on fetal weight, or congenital anomalies. In some species, such as the rabbit, conceptuses can be expelled during gestation (abortion) as a result of the death of the conceptuses or excessive maternal toxicity.

Two categories of congenital anomalies (alterations) are malformations and variations. Malformations tend to occur at low incidences, have a major impact on the animal, and are irreversible whereas variations are not. There are congenital anomalies for which there is no unanimous agreement on the classification as a

Table 9.1 Selected terminology for reproductive toxicity reports

Preferred term	Alternative term	Definition
Cohabitation	Cohousing Mating Pairing	Period during which males and females are housed together until evidence of mating is detected
Conceptus	Embryo Fetus Implant	An embryo or fetus
Developmental toxicity		Any adverse effect induced prior to adult life
Embryo		Conceptus from fertilization until closure of the hard palate
Embryofetal toxicity	Fetotoxicity	An adverse effect on the conceptus typically induced during organogenesis

Table 9.1 *continued*

Preferred term	Alternative term	Definition
Embryotoxicity	Embryolethality	An adverse effect on the conceptus induced during the embryonic period of development
Fertilization	Conception	Combination of sperm and egg
Fetus		Conceptus from closure of the hard palate until parturition
Gametogenesis, spermatogenesis, oogenesis		Production and maturation of the gametes
Gestation	Pregnancy	Period during which dam is pregnant
Implantation		Attachment of embryo to inner wall of uterus
Lactating female	Dam Mother	Dam with nursing pups
Litter		All conceptuses or pups from one dam
Mated	Bred Successful copulation	Female with evidence of mating (seminal plug or sperm in vagina, sometimes vaginal plug in cage tray); also confusingly used to refer to cohabitation
Parturition	Birth	
Postimplantation loss		Death of embryo or fetus after implantation
Postnatal	Lactation	The period after birth when referring to the offspring
Postpartum	Lactation Postparturition	The period after birth when referring to the dam
Pregnant female	Dam Gravid female Mother	Female with embryos or fetuses *in utero*
Preimplantation loss		Embryos dying prior to implantation, commonly expressed as corpora lutea – implants or this difference expressed as a percentage of corpora lutea
Pup	F_1 (F_2) generation Newborn Offspring Young	Rodent offspring prior to sexual maturation
Resorption rate	Fetal wastage Postimplantation loss Uterine death Uterine mortality	The incidence of reabsorbing dead conceptuses; can be subdivided into early or late depending on morphological criteria
Teratogen		An agent which induces structural malformations
Weaning		Separation of the offspring from the mother

malformation or a variation (e.g. wavy rib and supernumerary rib). Furthermore, there are sites of incomplete ossification which typically indicate delayed development.

Early workers in the field then known as "teratology" focused on the study of congenital malformations. Malformations had (and have) a tremendous clinical and social impact, much more than, for example, abortions, which are frequently undetected. This emphasis on malformations was reinforced by the thalidomide tragedy in which thousands of children were born with severely debilitating drug-induced congenital defects. Thus, embryofetal toxicity (Segment II) studies were for decades referred to as "teratology studies" and the focus was on detecting teratogens, i.e. agents which induce malformations.

More recently, there has been increased emphasis on other endpoints of embryofetal toxicity studies in addition to malformations: fetal weight, embryofetal death, and defects not considered to be malformations. This change reflects the recognition of several points. The first is that embryofetal death is a severe outcome which may have resulted from malformation. Since drug-induced developmental effects can vary from species to species, this may indicate a potential for causing malformation in other species. Secondly, it is now clear that malformations in animal models can occur secondarily to maternal toxicity and are therefore not all "teratogenic" responses necessarily indicating a severe hazard for humans. Thirdly, the induction of, or the increase in, the incidence of "variations" by a test compound, though not a "teratogenic" response, can nevertheless indicate a serious perturbation of development. Finally, there is no universal agreement on the definition of "teratogen". Thus, to avoid confusion one should refer to embryofetal toxicity or developmental toxicity rather than teratogenicity; however, a perspective on the risk should be provided on the nature of a particular adverse developmental finding.

Treatment in an embryofetal toxicity study approximately coincides with the period of major organogenesis, and examination of the uterine contents occurs at the end of gestation. The timing of the induction of toxic effects observed at the end of gestation can sometimes be inferred from the type of effect. For example, malformations of the cardiovascular system or early resorptions can only be induced during the embryonic period, and therefore the toxicity can be referred to as embryotoxicity. Often, however, it cannot be inferred whether the toxic insult occurred during the embryonic or fetal period. For example, it is usually not possible to conclude when decreases in fetal weight were induced or whether late resorptions occurred at the end of the embryonic period or the beginning of the fetal period. Even if it is clear that fetuses died late, just before study termination, the lethal insult may have occurred during the embryonic period. Thus, the term "fetotoxicity" cannot correctly be used in reference to an embryofetal toxicity study unless additional studies are conducted. For these reasons, it is common to refer to effects on the conceptus observed at the end of gestation as "embryofetal toxicity" or "developmental toxicity".

9.2.4 Pre- and Postnatal Toxicity

Since development, particularly of the brain, continues during the early postnatal period and, since effects induced during gestation and lactation can be expressed in F_1 adults, adverse effects observed during the postnatal period can appropriately be referred to as "developmental toxicity". For example, retardation of growth, delayed development of reflexes and developmental landmarks, and aberrations in behavioral tests can all be considered developmental toxicity when induced in a pre- and postnatal toxicity study in which treatment begins at implantation and continues through the lactation period (see Study Definitions below). When describing adverse developmental effects clearly induced during gestation in this type of study (e.g. effects observed in newborns), one provides more specific information by using the term "embryofetal toxicity" rather than "developmental toxicity" to refer to them.

9.2.5 Multiple Phases and Generations

Writing reports for fertility studies and pre- and postnatal toxicity studies is complicated (compared with general toxicity studies) by having multiple phases and generations. For example, in the fertility study, there are precohabitation, cohabitation, and gestation phases for the parental (F_0) generation and two generations: F_0 adults and F_1 fetuses. In the pre- and postnatal toxicity study, there are the gestation and postpartum (lactation) phases for the F_0 females and the preweaning, postweaning, cohabitation, gestation, and, in some cases, postpartum (lactation) portions of the postnatal period for the F_1 generation. Many of the parameters measured are specific to a particular phase and generation. In the fertility study, one or both sexes may have been treated. When both males and females are treated and cohabited in a ratio of 1:1, the results for fertility and mating performance for the two sexes will obviously be identical.

9.2.6 Study Definitions

For detailed design requirements for reproductive toxicity studies, the relevant regulatory guidelines should be consulted. In general, such studies should involve the exposure of sexually mature adults and all developmental stages (gametogenesis and conception to sexual maturity). The combined results from these studies give an overview of the immediate and delayed effects following administration of a compound throughout one complete life cycle (conception to conception in two generations). For convenience, the reproductive cycle is broken down into multiple phases, and studies designed to assess reproductive toxicity should ensure that compound administration covers all the phases shown in Table 9.2, as recommended in guidelines. Typically, these phases are combined into three or four studies based on the guidelines of the International Conference on Harmonization. These guidelines replaced similar guidelines which had specified three study types based on dosing period, which were referred to as Segment I, Segment II and Segment III studies. The new standard study types are briefly described below.

Fertility and early embryonic development (formerly "Segment I")

This study assesses toxicity resulting from treatment of males and females prior to and through mating, up to implantation. Estrus cycle, tubal transport,

Table 9.2 Phases of the reproductive cycle

Stage	Reproductive phase
A	Premating to conception
B	Conception to implantation
C	Implantation to closure of the hard palate
D	Closure of the hard palate to end of pregnancy
E	Birth to weaning
F	Weaning to sexual maturity

implantation and early preimplantation embryonic development are assessed in females. Functional defects on male reproductive organs not normally detected by histopathological examination are assessed in males.

Separate male and female fertility studies are often performed (cohabitation with non-treated animals) to identify clearly sex-specific toxicity.

Embryofetal development (formerly "Segment II")

The aim of this study is to detect adverse effects in the pregnant female and in embryofetal development after administration of the compound to pregnant females from implantation to closure of the hard palate. Endpoints include maternal toxicity and effects on embryofetal mortality, growth and development.

Pre- and postnatal development (formerly "Segment III")

This study is designed to detect the effects of treatment from implantation through weaning on the pregnant and lactating female and on the conceptus and offspring up to sexual maturity, including assessment of reproductive performance. The treatment period is a combination of those used previously in the Segment II and Segment III studies; however, the endpoints evaluated are only those included in the former Segment III studies.

·9.3 Report Outline

In general, it is clearest to have separate sections in both the Materials and Methods and the Results to describe each phase within each generation and, in the fertility study, to separate F_0 males and females when applicable. Thus, in a generalized outline form applicable to any study design including treatment of both sexes, both the Materials and Methods and Results sections would be organized as shown below.

I. F_0 Generation
   A. Mortality
   B. Clinical signs
   C. Body weight and food consumption
   D. Precoital interval, mating and fertility indices and pregnancy rate

E.   Gestation length and observations at parturition
F.   Necropsy
   1.   Males (including sperm motility and count)
   2.   Non-mated females
   3.   Caesarean section females
      a.   Maternal observations
      b.   Corpora lutea, implantations and pre-implantation loss
      c.   Post-implantation loss and litter size
      d.   Fetal weight and sex ratio
      e.   Fetal examination
   4.   Dams on Day 21 postpartum
      a.   Maternal observations
      b.   Implantations and post-implantation loss

II. F_1 Generation
  A.   Mortality
    1.   Pup data at birth
    2.   Preweaning
    3.   Postweaning
  B.   Clinical signs
  C.   Body weights
    1.   Pup data at birth and preweaning
    2.   Postweaning
  D.   Developmental tests
    1.   Physical development
    2.   Functional development
    3.   Behavioral development
  E.   Precoital interval, mating and fertility indices and pregnancy rate
  F.   Gestation length and observations at parturition
  G.   Necropsy
    1.   Day 56 ± 3
    2.   Males selected for reproductive performance
    3.   Non-pregnant females
    4.   Mated females which littered
       a.   Maternal observation
       b.   Implantation and post-implantation loss

III. F_2 Generation
  A.   Mortality
  B.   Clinical signs
  C.   Body weights
  D.   Terminal necropsy

Obviously, sections that do not apply to a particular study would be omitted.

9.4 Methods Sections

Methods sections should be kept as simple as possible. The sequence of topics should reflect the order described in Section 9.3, which approximates the chronological order of the study. Some writers may elect to use an outline form to simplify reader reference to specific elements of the methods used.

9.5 Results Sections

9.5.1 General Issues

The sequence of topics should reflect the order described in Section 9.3, which order will also be reproduced in the Methods section. The Results section should focus on presenting the findings, classifying the relationship of the findings to treatment (treatment-related, not treatment-related, or of uncertain relationship to treatment) and then justifying those classifications. When treatment-related findings or findings of uncertain relationship to treatment are not considered toxicologically significant, the reasons should be given.

Consistent with the policy of making it easy for the reader to find key information, each paragraph should begin with a topical sentence summarizing the major conclusions contained in the paragraph. This is different from writing a manuscript for publication, for which one builds an argument by making several points and then reaching a conclusion. In a report, the conclusions are given first, where they are easiest to find by the reader, and then the supporting arguments are given. For example: "There were statistically significant ($p \leqslant 0.05$), treatment-related lower body weight gains in the 30 and 100 mg/kg/day groups (-11% and -18%, respectively) compared with the control during the first 2 weeks of the study. Thereafter body weight gain was similar to control. There was no effect on body weight gain at 10 mg/kg/day."

In some more complicated cases, it may be advantageous to have a second paragraph describing the findings for a particular parameter. For example, when there is a treatment effect at the high dose and a finding of uncertain relationship to treatment in the middle dose, the first paragraph can describe the findings at the high dose and then a new paragraph could consider the middle-dose findings. This second paragraph could begin with the topical sentence summarizing the position concerning the middle-dose group and then elaborate on the arguments on both sides: "Body weight gain at 30 mg/kg/day during Weeks 1 through 4 was 8% lower compared with the controls and is considered to be of uncertain relationship to treatment. While a part of an apparent dose response, this was largely attributable to lower body weight gain in 2 animals and was not statistically significant ($p > 0.05$)". Also, in some cases where questionable findings are not considered treatment-related, the reasons to support the interpretation should be provided: these may include an absence of a dose response, similar historical control values, or the restriction of the findings to only a few animals.

An interpretation is most convincing if it is presented when the corresponding data are first described. The immediate interpretation does not leave the reader wondering what the writer's interpretation of the data is and may prevent the reader from reaching incorrect interpretations. Thus, when an observation is first mentioned, it should be made clear whether the finding is considered to be treatment-related, not treatment-related, or of uncertain relationship to treatment. Avoid reporting increases or decreases in a particular parameter without making it immediately clear whether the changes are considered to be treatment-related.

When describing findings, provide information about the severity of the effect. Provide quantitative information whenever practical. For example, "12% decrease in body weight gain" is preferable to "slight decrease in body weight gain". When percentages are not applicable, provide data such as "there was a 78 g body weight loss in the 100 mg/kg/day group compared with a 220 g increase in the control group".

9.5.2 Litter Data

The litter is the unit of treatment (via the dam) and therefore must be considered when discussing and interpret litter data. Statistical analyses on incidences of congenital anomalies are typically conducted on the percentage of litters affected (litter incidence) or on the proportion of fetuses affected (e.g. the percentage of fetuses affected within each litter). These are referred to as the litter and fetal incidences, respectively, and can be defined in the Methods section. The fetal incidence is often a more sensitive indicator of toxic effects than the litter incidence. Typical descriptions of findings are shown below:

- "There were no effects of treatment observed during the external, visceral and skeletal examinations of fetuses."
- "There was a treatment-related higher incidence of cleft palate in the 100 mg/kg/day group (7 fetuses from 3 of 21 litters compared with 0 fetuses among 23 litters in the control group)."
- "There was a dose-related higher incidence of supernumerary rib in the 30 and 100 mg/kg/day groups (fetal incidences of 17% and 28%, respectively) compared with the control (11%), which was statistically significant ($p \leqslant 0.05$) and considered treatment-related."
- "A low incidence of cleft palate in the 100 mg/kg/day group (2 fetuses from 2 of 21 litters) compared with control (0 fetuses from 23 litters) was not considered treatment-related, since no fetuses with cleft palate were observed in a previous study at that dosage level (PP 96-123) and equal or higher incidences have commonly been observed in historical control groups."

9.5.3 Relationship between Maternal and Developmental Toxicity

An agent which causes developmental toxicity at dosage levels which are not maternally toxic is referred to as a selective developmental toxin. More often, developmental toxicity occurs only at maternally toxic dosage levels. In this situation, it is of interest to know if the developmental toxicity is a result of a direct effect on the conceptus (direct developmental toxin) or is secondary to maternal toxicity (indirect developmental toxin). This is usually very difficult to demonstrate conclusively. However, it should be possible to determine if the developmental toxicity occurred primarily in those animals with the most severe maternal toxicity, i.e. when the developmental toxicity was correlated with the maternal toxicity. Depending on the outcome of this analysis, the following sorts of statements could be made to describe the relationship between the maternal and developmental toxicities.

- "The developmental toxicity occurred only in association with maternal toxicity."
- "The developmental toxicity occurred only at high, maternally toxic dosage levels and was of the type typically induced by maternal toxicity. Therefore, the test compound is not considered a developmental hazard."
- "The observation that the developmental toxicity occurred only in animals with the most severe maternal toxicity suggests that the developmental toxicity was secondary to the maternal toxicity."

9.6 Summary, Discussion and Conclusion sections

In the Summary, Discussion and Conclusion portions of the reports, it is important to separate the discussion of effects into the following categories, specifying the no observed effect level ("NOEL") for each:

1 F_0 males
   a. Effects on fertility and mating performance (with "reproductive" NOEL)
   b. Other toxic effects (with NOEL)
2 F_0 females
   a. Effects on fertility and mating performance (with "reproductive" NOEL)
   b. Other toxic effects (with NOEL)
3 Developmental toxicity (with NOEL).

Toxicologically significant findings are summarized in the Conclusion section and placed in the appropriate perspective. For example, the observed toxicity may reflect exaggerated pharmacological activity, may be expected for that class of compounds, or the species used in the study may be particularly sensitive to the test compound or the class of test compounds.

The Conclusion section should be as simple as possible. Avoid speculation. Refer to other studies, other compounds and literature references only as essential to support the arguments made. Raise issues only if pertinent to the safety assessment of the test compound. Ideally, each report should stand alone. One exception is when the selection of dosage levels has been based on a previous study in which case the basis for dosage selection is mentioned in the report for the subsequent study. Another exception is when studies have been repeated to confirm or refute previous findings. In this case, the overall interpretations made in each report should be based on all of the data with references between the studies as necessary. The conclusions of the two studies should agree.

In the Summary, state the purpose of the study. Briefly describe the study design in text form. Summarize the results in a manner similar to that in the Conclusion section. Findings that are dismissed in the Results or Conclusion sections as being not treatment-related or not toxicologically significant need not be mentioned in the Summary.

10

Example of a General Toxicology Report

G. J. NOHYNEK

Rhône-Poulenc Rorer, Vitry sur Seine, France

M. Y. WELLS

Rhône-Poulenc Rorer, Drug Safety Department, Vitry sur Seine, France

R. J. SZOT

Consultant in Toxicology, Flemington, NJ, USA

and S. GOSSELIN

ITR Laboratories Canada Inc., Montreal, Canada

PP 27567: 3-Month Oral Toxicity in Sprague-Dawley Rats

Dose levels: 5, 25, 125 mg/kg/day

Study Number: PP 94-0112

Contents

PP 27567: 3-Month Oral Toxicity in Sprague-Dawley Rats

Study Number: PP 94-0112

Summary

The purpose of this study was to assess the oral toxicity of PP 27567, a systemic inhibitor of acetyl-CoA:cholesterol acyltransferase (ACAT). Four groups of 20 male and 20 female Sprague–Dawley rats received daily oral doses of 0 (control), 5, 25 or 125 mg/kg PP 27567 for 3 months. Satellite groups of 6 males and 6 females per dosage level were included for determination of plasma drug levels. Parameters evaluated included clinical signs of toxicity, body weight and food consumption, plasma drug levels on days 1 and 88 of dosing at 2, 6, 10 and 24 hours after compound administration, mid-study and terminal hematology, clinical chemistry, urinalysis, organ weights, necropsy observations and histopathologic examination of principal tissues.

Plasma drug concentrations were dose-related, higher in females than in males, and similar on days 1 and 88. Maximal values were observed at 2 (5 or 25 mg/kg/day) or 6 (125 mg/kg/day) hours after administration (range of c_{Max} values at 125 mg/kg/day on day 1 was 6.1 to 11.4 μg/ml in males, and 8.2 to 12.5 μg/ml in females). No compound-related mortality occurred during the study. Clinical signs of dose-related severity and incidence were limited to groups receiving 25 or 125 mg/kg/day and consisted of reduced motor activity, chromodacryorrhea and ptosis. PP 27567 produced a dose-related decrease in mean body weight as compared with control values, which was moderate (-7% and -10% in males and females, respectively) at 25 mg/kg/day and marked (-16% and -19% in males and females, respectively) at 125 mg/kg/day, and which correlated with a lower food consumption at these dose levels. Compound-related clinical pathology changes at 125 mg/kg/day included higher RBC parameters, changes in mean electrolyte values, higher ALAT and ASAT (max. 3.2-fold and 3.0-fold, respectively) values, slightly higher plasma cholesterol (females only) and mean urinary volume. Changes at 25 mg/kg/day were limited to minimal increases in ALAT and ASAT. Clinical pathology values at 5 mg/kg/day were comparable with those of control groups. At 125 mg/kg/day the mean liver weight was higher than that in controls, adrenal and testis weights were lower; these weight differences correlated histologically with periportal hepatocellular hypertrophy, degeneration and atrophy of the adrenal cortex, and atrophy of the seminiferous tubules of the testes. Changes at 25 mg/kg/day were limited to slightly higher mean liver weights, associated with mild periportal hepatocellular hypertrophy. Organ weights in the groups receiving 5 mg/kg/day were unaffected, and no compound-related histopathologic changes were observed in this group.

In conclusion, oral administration of 125 mg/kg/day PP 27567 for 3 months affected the adrenals, liver and testis. A dose of 25 mg/kg/day produced mild changes in the liver. No adverse effects were noted at 5 mg/kg/day.

Report Signatures

TESTING FACILITY: SPONSOR:

Name: Name:

Address: Address:

STUDY DIRECTOR: _____

                       Name, Qualification(s), Position, Date

PATHOLOGIST: _____

                       Name, Qualification(s), Position, Date

OTHER AUTHOR(S):   _____

                       Name, Qualification(s), Position, Date

APPROVED BY[1]:   _____

                       Name, Qualification(s), Position, Date

[1]Management Approval

Introduction

PP 27567 is a systemic inhibitor of acetyl-CoA:cholesterol acyltransferase (ACAT) which is developed for treatment of hypercholesterolemia in man. The purpose of this study was to assess the oral toxicity of PP 27567 when administered in daily doses to Sprague–Dawley rats for 3 months.

In a previous 1-month oral study in rats which used dose levels of 25, 125 or 500 mg/kg/day (Report PP 93-0063; 1993), a dose of 500 mg/kg/day produced marked clinical signs, a markedly lower body weight (-20% in females at study termination, compared with control mean) associated with lower food consumption, and adverse changes in the adrenal gland (marked atrophy of all layers of the cortex), testis (reduced testis weights, diffuse testicular degeneration) and the liver (markedly higher liver weight, fatty changes, periportal hypertrophy). Effects at 125 mg/kg/day were limited to a minimally lower body weight, and mild to moderate changes in the adrenals, testes and liver. A dose of 25 mg/kg/day produced a minimally higher liver weight only.

Therefore, considering the longer duration of administration in the present study, 125 mg/kg/day was considered an appropriate high-dose level. The low and intermediate doses of 5 and 25 mg/kg/day were selected to establish a dose–response relationship for potential adverse effects of PP 27567.

Materials and Methods

Male and female Sprague-Dawley rats (Charles River France) were used in this study. At the start of the study, the animals were 53–55 days old and their mean body weights were 225 and 182 grams for males and females, respectively. Three groups of 20 male and 20 female rats were treated orally (esophageal intubation) with PP 27567 at daily dose levels of 5, 25 or 125 mg/kg for 90 or 91 consecutive days. PP 27567 was suspended in a 0.5% aqueous solution of methylcellulose. The volume of administration was 3 ml/kg. Groups of 20 male and 20 female rats were kept as controls and received the vehicle. Satellite groups consisting of 5 males and 5 females per dose level were included in this study for determination of plasma drug levels on days 1 and 88, at 2, 6, 10 and 24 hours after compound administration. After collection of the last blood sample, these animals were sacrificed but not necropsied. During the treatment period, the animals of the main groups were observed daily for clinical signs and weighed weekly. Their food and water consumption was measured weekly. Blood samples were collected from treated animals on day 44 (males) or 45 (females) for determination of interim clinical chemistry or hematology values. Approximately 24 hours following the last treatment, blood samples were collected for terminal clinical chemistry and hematology analysis. On day 90 (males) or 91 (females), the animals were sacrificed by carbon dioxide inhalation and necropsied. The weight of principal organs was determined, and principal tissues were processed for histopathologic examination. Details of the materials and methods used in this study are provided in Appendix II of this report.

Results

*1 **Plasma Drug Analysis*** (see individual and summary values, pages 000 and 000)

The magnitude of the observed plasma concentrations indicated that PP 27567 was well absorbed after oral administration. Plasma concentrations of PP 27567 were dose-related, approximately proportional to the administered dose, and higher in females than in males. Values measured on day 88 of the study were comparable with those observed after the first dose. Maximal values (c_{Max}) which were recorded in the 125 mg/kg/day group 2 or 6 hours after administration were in the range shown in Table 1.

The concentration/time curves for the plasma levels of PP 27567 on day 1 and day 88 are displayed in Figures 1 and 2.

Table 1 PP 27567: 3-Month oral toxicity study in rats. Range of maximal plasma concentrations (c_{Max}/ μg/ml) on study days 1 and 88.

| | c_{Max} (μg/ml) | | | |
| | Day 1 | | Day 88 | |
Dose (mg/kg/day)	Males	Females	Males	Females
5	<0.05^a–0.42	0.81–1.13	<0.05–0.25	0.65–0.84
25	1.42–2.36	3.58–4.21	0.85–1.45	2.45–3.95
125	6.13–11.42	8.23–12.5	3.05–6.40	5.45–10.12

^{a}Limit of quantification of the analytical method

Table 2 PP 27567: 3-Month oral toxicity in rats. Mean AUC_{0-24h} values (μg.h/ml) on days 1 and 88.

Dose (mg/kg)	Day 1 (males)	Day 1 (females)	Day 88 (males)	Day 88 (females)
5	2.6	6.9	2.3	5.38
25	18.3	28.4	10.5	17.3
125	86.5	130.1	76.2	148.7

At 24 hours after doses of 5 or 25 mg/kg/day, plasma concentrations of PP 27567 were generally below the limit of detection of the analytical method. At 125 mg/kg/day, approximately 1.9 to 3.9 μg/ml of the compound was present in the plasma for 24 hours after administration.

Mean AUC values were higher in females than in males. AUC values on Days 1 and 88 were comparable and increased in approximate proportion to the administered dose as shown in Table 2.

2 In-life Observations/Measurements

2.1 Mortality (see page 000, necropsy observations)

No compound-related mortality was observed during this study. Two male animals (No. 402, 125 mg/kg/day and No. 315, 25 mg/kg/day) and one female animal (No. 807, 125 mg/kg/day) were found dead on study days 28, 65 and 81, respectively. Necropsy findings (congested lungs, traces of white particles in the bronchi) suggested that these deaths were caused by dosing accidents. One female (No. 713, 25 mg/kg/day) was found prostrate on day 70, had a stained anogenital region and lost weight on the two subsequent days. Because of its deteriorating clinical condition, this animal was sacrificed for ethical reasons on day 72 of the study. Although the cause of the poor condition of the animal was undetermined (see Pathology section of this report, page 000), it was not considered to be related to PP 27567 since it was an isolated incident at the mid-dose level.

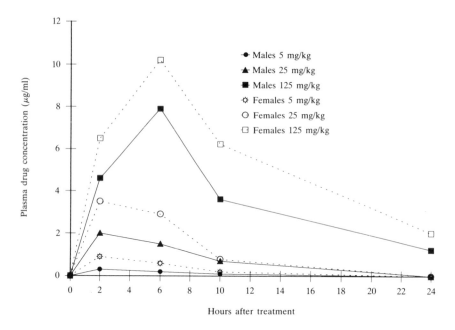

Figure 1   PP 27567: 3-Month oral toxicity study in rats. Mean plasma drug concentrations (μg/ml) at 5, 25 and 125 mg/kg/day. Values on day 1.

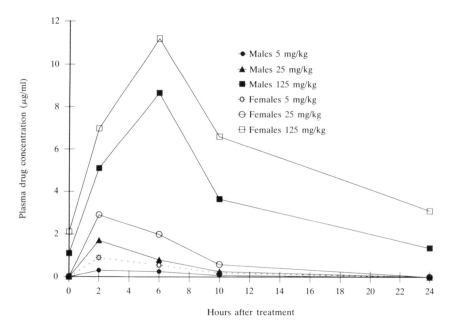

Figure 2   PP 27567: 3-Month oral toxicity study in rats. Mean plasma drug concentrations (μg/ml) at 5, 25 and 125 mg/kg/day. Values on day 88.

2.2 Clinical signs (see pages 000–000)

Compound-related clinical signs were noted from week 2 through the end of the study in all animals receiving 125 mg/kg/day and from week 15 to study termination in some female animals receiving 25 mg/kg/day. The incidence and the severity of these signs were dose-related and were generally more severe in females than in males; they consisted of reduced motor activity and ptosis (all animals at 125 mg/kg/day and 3/20 to 6/20 females at 25 mg/kg/day) and chromodacryorrhea (3/20 to 5/20 females at 125 mg/kg/day). Most animals at 125 mg/kg/day had a rough hair coat during the last weeks of the study. No compound-related clinical signs were noted at 5 mg/kg/day. With the exception of the prostration observed in female No. 713, 25 mg/kg/day (see Subsection 2.1), all other signs/observations recorded during this study are commonly observed in our laboratory and were not attributed to PP 27567.

2.3 Body weight (see table on page 000, and individual results, pages 000–000)

Administration of PP 27567 affected the mean body weight in groups receiving 25 or 125 mg/kg/day as shown in Table 3.

At 125 mg/kg/day, lower mean body weights became apparent in male and female groups after 3 weeks of treatment. The difference in body weight increased progressively during the course of the study, reached statistical significance after 4 weeks and resulted in markedly lower mean body weight at the end of the study. Similar, but milder effects on body weight were noted in the groups receiving 25 mg/kg/day; the difference reached statistical significance only during the final 3 weeks of the study. At 5 mg/kg/day, minimal effects on body weight were noted at the end of the study. Although this difference may be related to the administration of PP 27567, it was slight (-2% and -4% compared with control means in males and females, respectively) and within the range of the common variation of this parameter, and was therefore considered to be of no toxicological significance.

Table 3 PP 27567: 3-Month oral toxicity in rats. Mean body weight on days 32, 65 and 89 of the study (percentage change compared with control mean values).

Dose (mg/kg/day)	Sex	Day 32	Day 65	Day 89
5	M	—[a]	—	-2%
	F	—	-2%	-4%
25	M	—	-4%	-7%
	F	-2%	-6%	-10%*
125	M	-9%	-13%*	-16%*
	F	-12%*	-19%*	-19%*

$*p < 0.05$
[a]No effect

Table 4: PP 27567: 3-Month oral toxicity in rats. Mean weekly food consumption in Weeks 5, 9 and 12 of the study (percentage change compared with control mean values).

Dose (mg/kg/day)	Sex	Week 5	Week 9	Week 12
5	M	—[a]	—	—
	F	—	—	−4%
25	M	—	−2%	−4%
	F	—	−4%	−8%*
125	M	−2%	−6%*	−11%*
	F	−5%*	−9%*	−14%*

*$p < 0.05$
[a] No change, compared with control means

2.4 *Food and water consumption* (see tables, pages 000–000 and individual results on pages 000–000)

A compound- and dose-related lower food consumption which was correlated with the reduction in body weight was noted in all groups receiving PP 27567 at 25 or 125 mg/kg/day. Mean values are shown in Table 4.

Treatment with PP 27567 resulted in a dose-related lower mean food consumption when compared with control means. Female rats appeared somewhat more affected than males. At 125 mg/kg/day, lower food consumption became apparent in male and female groups during the fifth week of treatment. The difference in food consumption between the groups receiving 125 mg/kg/day and the control groups became progressively more marked during the course of the study and reached statistical significance from week 12 until the end of the study. Similar, but milder effects on food consumption were noted in the groups receiving 25 mg/kg/day; these reached statistical difference in females during the final weeks of the study. At 5 mg/kg/day, minimally decreased food consumption, which occurred only in females during the final weeks of the study, remained within the range of the common variation of this parameter and was considered to be of no toxicological significance. Water consumption was unaffected by treatment.

2.5 *Ophthalmology* (see individual results, pages 000–000)

Remnants of hyaloid vessels or a noticeable suture line of the anterior cortex of the lens were observed during the pre-study examination and on day 30 in some control animals and in some animals at 125 mg/kg/day. These vestigial fetal structures were no longer noted at the end of the study and were attributed to the young age of the animals. Small opalescent vesicles were observed in the superficial part of the corneal stroma in some male animals of the control, the 125 mg/kg/day and 5 mg/kg/day groups. This lesion was diagnosed as corneal dystrophy. Some minor changes were noted in the nucleus of the lens in a few animals of the control, 5 and 25 mg/kg/day groups. A similar incidence of these lesions has been reported for Sprague–Dawley rats of this strain and age (Taradach and Greaves, 1984). Because these changes were not dose-related in incidence, and since the incidence of these changes remained within our historical control range, they were considered to be of spontaneous origin.

3 Clinical Pathology

3.1 Hematology (see summary and individual values, pages 000–000 and 000–000)

At 125 mg/kg/day in both sexes, the administration of PP 27567 was associated with increases in RBC count, hemoglobin and hematocrit (+18%, when compared with control mean values). This effect correlated with electrolyte imbalances and increased urinary volume, and indicates hemoconcentration.

3.2 Clinical chemistry (see summary and individual values, pages 000–000 and 000–000)

Compound-related changes included electrolyte abnormalities, higher mean ALAT and ASAT values in both sexes and increases in cholesterol in females only, as compared with mean control values. Markedly higher serum K^+ and moderately lower serum Na^+ and Cl^- were observed at 125 mg/kg/day. Mean values are displayed in Table 5.

Mild increases in ALAT (maximum 3.2-fold and 2.5-fold of control means in males and females, respectively) and ASAT (maximum 3-fold and 2.2-fold in males and females, respectively) were observed at 25 and 125 mg/kg/day. A slightly higher mean cholesterol value (+36%) was observed in females only at 125 mg/kg/day. Slightly higher urea and lower total protein, albumin and albumin/globulin ratio in both sexes were associated with administration of 125 mg/kg/day PP 27567. These changes may be secondary to the decreased food consumption observed at this dose level.

Other compound-associated variations in clinical chemistry parameters were within the limits of our reference range data, were slight in magnitude and/or displayed no trends which were attributable to compound administration.

Table 5 PP 27567: 3-Month oral toxicity study in rats. Mean serum electrolyte changes on day 90 at 125 mg/kg/day.

Parameter	Sex	Results[a]
Na^+	male	−11% *
	female	−13% *
K^+	male	+38%
	female	−51% *
Cl^-	male	−9%
	female	−12% *

$^*p \leqslant 0.05$
[a]Percentage change compared with control mean values

3.3 Urinalysis (see summary and individual values, pages 000 and 000)

Compound-related effects were limited to increased mean urinary volume in the 125 mg/kg/day rats (+38% in males; +55% in females), when compared with control means.

4 Anatomic Pathology

4.1 Organ weights (see summary and individual values, pages 000 and 000–000)

Treatment with PP 27567 was associated with slightly lower mean absolute and relative adrenal weights at 125 mg/kg/day (both sexes), dose-related, slightly higher mean absolute and relative liver weights at 25 and 125 mg/kg/day (both sexes), and lower absolute and relative testis weights in males treated at 125 mg/kg/day. These findings are summarized in Table 6.

Table 6. PP 27576: 3-Month oral toxicity study in rats. Compound-related absolute and relative organ weight changes (percentage) compared with controls.

	Males			Females		
Dose (mg/kg/day)	5	25	125	5	25	125
Adrenal	NT	NT	−8 (−4)	NT	NT	−13 (−5)
Liver	NT	+10 (+8)	+21* (+18*)	NT	+12 (+11)	+25* (+22*)
Testes	NT	NT	−19* (−15)	NA	NA	NA

NA = not applicable; NT = no compound-related changes; *$p \leqslant 0.05$

There were no other compound-related organ weight findings. Slight variations between individual animals in both the absolute and relative organ weights, which had no relationship to dose or sex, and which sometimes achieved statistical significance, were observed but were considered incidental and unrelated to treatment with PP 27567.

4.2 Necropsy findings (see summary and individual values, pages 000–000 and 000–000)

Compound-related macroscopic findings consisted of bilateral small and soft testes in males treated at 125 mg/kg/day. All other macroscopic findings were incidental and typical of Sprague–Dawley rats of similar age. Three animals died prior to the termination of the study: two males and one female (M402, 125 mg/kg/day; M315, 25 mg/kg/day; F807, 125 mg/kg/day) which were found dead on study days 28, 65 and 81, respectively, and had gross and microscopic findings which suggested that their deaths were related to gavage accidents (pulmonary congestion and hemorrhage, foreign material in trachea, bronchi and alveoli). The cause of the deteriorating condition of the female (F713, 25 mg/kg/day) which was killed for ethical reasons (day 72) was not determined by either gross or microscopic examination. However, its deteriorating condition was not considered related to treatment with PP 27567, because of the lack of a dose relationship as well as its isolated incidence.

4.3 Histopathology (see summary and individual values, pages 000–000 and 000–000)

Treatment with PP 27567 was associated with degeneration and atrophy of the adrenal cortex at 125 mg/kg/day (both sexes), periportal hepatocellular hypertrophy and increased individual cell necrosis in the livers of rats (both sexes) at 25 and 125 mg/kg/day, and atrophy of the seminiferous tubules of the testes in males treated at 125 mg/kg/day.

In the adrenal gland, 12/20 males and 20/20 females treated at 125 mg/kg/day had mild to marked degeneration and necrosis of the zona fasciculata and zona reticularis, and mild atrophy of the zona glomerulosa. Degenerate cortical cells were characterized by decreased cell size, pyknotic nuclei and decreased lipid content. Other adrenocortical lesions included thickening of the capsule, multifocal mononuclear cell infiltrates, occasional cholesterol cleft formation, presence of hemosiderin pigments, and multifocal mineralization.

In the liver, 15/20 males and 17/20 females treated at 125 mg/kg/day had minimal to mild periportal hepatocellular hypertrophy. An increased incidence of individual cell necrosis in the liver observed at 25 and 125 mg/kg/day was interpreted to be an incidental finding since the lesions were minimal to mild in severity and were also observed in control animals.

In the testes, 12/20 males treated at 125 mg/kg/day had bilateral, mild to moderate, multifocal atrophy of the seminiferous tubules. This lesion was characterized by multifocal areas of seminiferous tubules which were either devoid of spermatozoa and/or immature sperm types or seminiferous tubules with germinal epithelium undergoing various stages of degeneration. In all cases, Sertoli cells, spermatogonia and the basement membrane in affected seminiferous tubules were intact and did not show evidence of degenerative changes. There were no other histopathologic findings related to treatment with PP 27567. All other microscopic findings were incidental or related to orbital venous plexus blood sampling and were typical of those lesions observed in Sprague-Dawley rats of similar age.

Discussion

The plasma drug levels, which were higher in females than in males, correlated with the adverse in-life effects (clinical signs, lower mean body weight and food consumption), which were generally more severe in females than in males. These findings confirm the results of a previous 1-month study which indicated that females are more affected by PP 27567 than males (Study PP/DS 93-0063). In the present study, clinical pathology, organ weight and histopathologic changes occurred at similar severity and incidence in both sexes. Moderately lower serum Na^+ and Cl^- and markedly elevated serum K^+ at 125 mg/kg/day correlated with atrophy in the adrenal cortex (zona glomerulosa), and were consistent with adrenal insufficiency. The higher mean urinary volume at this dose level is interpreted to be secondary to the loss of serum Na^+. Though the areas in the adrenal cortex which are responsible for the production of both mineralocorticoids and glucocorticoids were affected, no compound-related changes in serum glucose were noted in these animals. Lower mean absolute and relative adrenal weights at 125 mg/kg/day correlated with adrenal cortical degeneration (zona fascicularis and zona reticularis) and atrophy (zona glomerulosa). The adrenal cortical lesions were interpreted to be a primary cytotoxic effect of PP 27567, and were consistent with lesions reported with other ACAT inhibitors in the literature (Dominick *et al.*, 1993).

Mild increases in ALAT and ASAT at 25 and 125 mg/kg/day and a minimal increase in cholesterol in females only at 125 mg/kg/day correlated with higher absolute and relative liver weights at 25 and 125 mg/kg/day and periportal hepatocellular hypertrophy and a higher incidence of individual cell necrosis at 125 mg/kg/day. No microscopic changes in the liver were observed at 25 mg/kg/day. The periportal hypertrophy was interpreted to be an adaptive response of the liver to PP 27567, and was consistent with lesions reported with other ACAT inhibitors in the literature (Dominick *et al.*, 1993). Because individual cell necrosis was also found in control animals, and because it was minimal to mild in severity, this lesion was considered to be an incidental finding.

Lower mean absolute and relative testis weights at 125 mg/kg/day correlated with the small, soft testes seen at necropsy and the atrophy of the seminiferous tubules observed histopathologically in this dose group. This effect may be due to decreased testosterone production secondary to the perturbation of cholesterol metabolism in the Leydig cells of the testis and the zona reticularis of the adrenal cortex. These results are consistent with those found in an earlier reproduction study (Study No. PP 92-037, 1992), in which a lower fertility was observed in male rats.

Conclusion

Adverse in-life effects of oral administration of 125 mg/kg/day PP 27567 for 3 months were more severe in females than in males and included clinical signs, lower mean body weight and food consumption. The target organs were the adrenals, liver and testis. Administration of 25 mg/kg/day produced mild in-life effects and mild changes in the liver. No adverse effects were noted at 5 mg/kg/day.

References

Dominick M. A., McGuire E. J., Reindel J. F., Bobrowski W. F., Bocan T. M. A. and Gough A. W. (1993) Subacute toxicity of a novel inhibitor of Acyl-CoA: cholesterol acyltransferase in Beagle dogs. Fundamental and Applied Toxicology, 20; 217–224.

Report PP/DS 92-037 (1992) PP 27567: Oral Fertility Study in Male Sprague-Dawley Rats.

Report PP/DS 93-0063 (1993) PP 27567: 30-Day Oral Toxicity Study in Sprague-Dawley Rats.

Taradach C. and Greaves P. (1984) Spontaneous eye lesions in laboratory animals: incidence in relation to age. CRC Critical Reviews in Toxicology, 12; 121–147.

11

Example of a Reproductive Toxicology Report

G. COPPING

Rhône-Poulenc Rorer, Drug Safety Development, Vitry sur Seine, France

and R. L. CLARK

Rhône-Poulenc Rorer Research and Development, Drug Safety Department, Collegeville, USA

PP 27567: Oral one-generation reproductive toxicity study
in rats including F_1 reproductive performance

Dose levels: 3, 10, 30 mg/kg/day

Study Number: PP 93-1234

PP 27567: Oral one-generation reproductive toxicity study in rats including F_1 reproductive performance

R. Clark and G. Copping

The purpose of this study was to assess the effect of oral administration of PP 27567 upon gonadal function, mating behavior and fertility of male and female rats when treated in the F_0 generation, and to assess the subsequent development of the F_1 generation up to sexual maturity including mating to produce an F_2 generation.

Thirty-six Sprague-Dawley rats/sex/group (Crl:CDr(SD)BR), approximately 7 weeks (males) and 9 weeks (females) old at the beginning of treatment, were used. Animals in the control group received water, and animals in the treated groups received PP 27567 as an aqueous solution at dose levels of 3, 10 or 30 mg/kg/day by the oral route in a dosing volume of 2 ml/kg/day.

Only F_0 rats were treated: males for 28 days pre-pairing, throughout pairing and up to necropsy, and females for 14 days pre-pairing and throughout pairing, gestation and lactation. Observations included mortality, clinical examination, food consumption, body weight and macroscopic examination at necropsy. Twenty F_0 females per group were sacrificed on day 20 of gestation for examination of their uterine contents, including external, visceral and skeletal examination of fetuses. The remaining females were allowed to litter and rear their young to weaning on day 21 postpartum. The physical and functional development and behavior of the F_1 generation were evaluated on standardized litters. On postnatal day 58 ± 2, 1 male and 1 female per litter were selected for subsequent evaluation of reproductive performance following pairing and the observation of the F_2 generation up to postnatal day 7.

At 30 mg/kg/day, PP 27567 induced adverse parental effects including salivation, reduced food intake and body weight gain, slight reductions in fertility index and pregnancy rate, and a slight increase in gestation length. These effects were associated with mild effects in the F_1 generation, as indicated by lower mean fetal body weight, delayed fetal ossification, a slight decrease in birth index, and reduced pup body weight at birth and during the pre-weaning period.

At 10 mg/kg/day, with the exception of salivation in a few F_0 animals, no adverse effects were observed in the F_0, F_1 and F_2 generations.

At 3 mg/kg/day, no adverse effects were observed in the F_0, F_1 and F_2 generations.

In conclusion, the reproductive and developmental no-effect level of PP 27567 under the conditions of this study is 10 mg/kg/day.

Study chronology

F$_0$ parents

Dosing:	males	28 days pre-pairing, throughout pairing and up to necropsy
	females	14 days pre-pairing and throughout pairing, gestation and lactation
Necropsy:	males	after pairing period
	females	caesarean section groups: day 20 of gestation postnatal groups: day 21 postpartum

F$_1$ pups

Culling	day 4 postpartum (8 pups)
Weaning	day 21 postpartum

Developmental tests

Physical
- incisor eruption   from day 7 postpartum
- eye opening   from day 11 postpartum
- balano-preputial separation   from day 40 postpartum
- vaginal opening   from day 30 postpartum

Functional
- negative geotaxis   from day 4 postpartum
- auditory startle reflex   from day 10 postpartum
- pupillary reflex   on day 19 postpartum

Behavioral
- water maze – learning   day 42 ± 3 postpartum
          – memory   7 days after learning test
- open field exploratory   on day 49 ± 3 postpartum
and locomotor activities

Selection for pairing	day 58 ± 2 postpartum
Necropsy	day 58 ± 2 postpartum

F$_1$ parents

Pairing	21-day period from 69 to 83 days old
Necropsy: males	after pairing period
females	on day 8 ± 1 postpartum

F$_2$ pups

Culling	day 4 postpartum (8 pups)
Necropsy	day 8 ± 1 postpartum

1 Introduction

The purpose of this study was to assess the effect of oral administration of PP 27567 upon gonadal function, mating behavior and fertility in male and female rats, and to assess the subsequent development of the F_1 generation up to sexual maturity including mating to produce an F_2 generation. The dose levels selected were based on the results of an embryofetal developmental toxicity study in rats (Report PP 674, 1993) which indicated lower maternal body weight gain at 30 mg/kg/day associated with lower fetal weight, and the results of a 6-month oral toxicity study in rats (Report PP 711, 1993) which indicated that administration of 30 mg/kg/day produced a lower mean body weight gain in both males and females and a reduction in mean ovary weight and ovarian atrophy in females. The no-effect level was 10 mg/kg/day in the embryofetal developmental toxicity study and 3 mg/kg/day in the 6-month toxicity study. Based on these results, dose levels of 3, 10 and 30 mg/kg/day PP 27567 were selected.

2 Materials and Methods

Aqueous solutions of PP 27567 were administered by oral gavage to groups of 36 male and 36 female rats at daily dose levels of 3, 10 or 30 mg/kg/day. Males were treated for 28 days pre-pairing, throughout pairing and up to necropsy. Females were treated for 14 days pre-pairing and throughout pairing, gestation and lactation. A control group of 36 males and 36 females received the vehicle alone over the same periods. Observations included mortality, clinical examination, food consumption, body weight and macroscopic examination at necropsy.

Twenty F_0 females per group were euthanatized on day 20 of gestation for examination of their uterine contents, including external, visceral and skeletal examination of fetuses. The remaining females were allowed to litter and rear their young to weaning on day 21 postpartum. The physical and functional development and behavior of the F_1 generation were evaluated on standardized litters. Details of study protocol materials and methods are given in Appendix 1 of this report. On postnatal day 58 ± 2, 1 male and 1 female per litter were selected for subsequent evaluation of reproductive performance following pairing and the observation of the F_2 generation up to postnatal day 7.

3 Results and Discussion

3.1 *F_0 Generation*

3.1.1 *Mortality*

No compound-related mortality was observed in the F_0 generation.

One male (No. 3109, 10 mg/kg/day) was euthanatized for ethical reasons on day 36 of the pre-pairing period because of the presence of an abdominal and subcutaneous mass which was observed from day 19.

Two females (No. 3307, 10 mg/kg/day and No. 3357, 30 mg/kg/day) were euthanatized for procedural reasons (litter less than six pups) on days 4 and 6 postpartum. No macroscopic findings were noted in these animals at necropsy.

3.1.2 Clinical signs

At 30 and 10 mg/kg/day, compound-related clinical signs were limited to salivation observed immediately after treatment. This sign was recorded from the first week of treatment up to the end of the treatment period in both sexes. The incidence and frequency of salivation were dose-related.

All other clinical signs monitored during the treatment period were not considered to be related to PP 27567.

No compound-related clinical signs were noted in animals treated at 3 mg/kg/day.

3.1.3 Body weight and food consumption

PP 27567 produced a treatment-related decrease in food intake and body weight gain at 30 mg/kg/day in males and females. Mean food consumption was less than that of controls at 30 mg/kg/day from the second week of treatment in males and from the first week of treatment in females. As a consequence, mean body weight gain during the dosing period (in males and females during pre-pairing and in females during gestation and lactation periods) was lower in this group (approximately −15% to −30% when compared with controls). These differences in food intake and mean body weight gain reached statistical significance during the pre-pairing (males and females) and gestation periods.

Slightly lower food consumption and body weight gain were noted at the end of the pre-pairing period in 10 mg/kg/day males.

There were no differences in group mean body weight and food consumption between the control and the 3 mg/kg/day groups.

3.1.4 Precoital interval, mating and fertility indices and pregnancy rate

Precoital interval and mating index were comparable in all groups.

Fertility indices and pregnancy rate were slightly lower at 30 mg/kg/day when compared with controls (22% and 19%, respectively). These reductions did not reach statistical significance.

No effects on fertility indices or pregnancy rate were observed at 10 and 3 mg/kg/day.

3.1.5 Gestation length· and observations at parturition

Gestation length and parturition index were similar in all groups and there were no signs of dystocia in any group.

At 30 mg/kg/day, gestation length was significantly but minimally higher (mean 22 ± 0.5 days compared with mean 21.5 ± 0.5 days) than that of controls, while birth index was slightly and non-significantly lower (−11% when compared with controls).

At 10 and 3 mg/kg/day, gestation length and birth index were similar to those of the controls.

3.1.6 Necropsy

3.1.6.1 Males
There were no treatment-related effects on mean sperm count, motility or vitality of spermatozoa.

Group mean relative testicular weight was significantly higher at 30 mg/kg/day when compared with controls. This increase was related to the significantly lower mean body weight observed in this group. Group mean absolute epididymal weight was significantly lower at 30 mg/kg/day when compared with controls. Group mean absolute and relative testicular and epididymal weights were comparable in the control, 10 and 3 mg/kg/day groups.

No compound-related macroscopic findings were noted at terminal necropsy.

3.1.6.2 Non-mated females
No compound-related macroscopic findings were noted at necropsy.

3.1.6.3 Caesarean section of mated females on day 20 of gestation
Maternal observations. No compound-related macroscopic findings were noted at terminal necropsy.

Corpora lutea, implantations and pre-implantation loss. Mean numbers of corpora lutea, implantations and pre-implantation loss were similar between the control and treated groups.

Post-implantation loss and litter size. Mean numbers of early and late uterine deaths and post-implantation loss were similar between the control and treated groups.

Fetal weight and sex ratio. Sex ratio was unaffected by treatment. Mean fetal weight was significantly lower at 30 mg/kg/day (-14% when compared with controls). This effect was considered likely to be secondary to decreased maternal food consumption and body weight. At 10 and 3 mg/kg/day, mean fetal weight was unaffected by treatment.

Fetal examination. External and internal observations revealed a range of malformations and variations in all groups. There was no indication of a compound-related trend in the type or incidence of these anomalies. At 30 mg/kg/day, there was a slight delay in skeletal ossification characterized by higher incidence of fetuses with incomplete or unossified supraoccipitals, exoccipitals, thoracic vertebral centra, sternebrae, pubis bones and hindpaw distal phalanges. These observations were consistent with the lower mean fetal weight secondary to lower maternal body weight observed at this dose level. At 10 and 3 mg/kg/day, skeletal examination of fetuses revealed a range of changes which were of a type or which occurred at an incidence similar to that of controls. There was no evidence of a teratogenic effect.

3.1.6.4 Dams on day 21 postpartum
Maternal observations. No compound-related macroscopic findings were noted at necropsy.

Implantations and post-implantation loss. At 30 mg/kg/day, the mean number of implantations observed on day 21 postpartum was slightly lower than the control value. As there was no equivalent effect observed in the caesarean section group, this was not considered to be compound-related. At 10 and 3 mg/kg/day, the mean number of implantations was comparable to that for controls. Mean post-implantation loss was comparable in all groups.

3.2 F_1 Generation

3.2.1 Mortality

3.2.1.1 Pup data at birth
In the 30 mg/kg/day group, mean litter size was significantly lower than the control value and was considered to be related to the lower number of implantations. Since such an effect was not observed in the caesarean section group or in previous embryofetal developmental toxicity studies (Reports PP 674 and PP 684, 1993), this was not considered to be compound-related. In the 10 and 3 mg/kg/day groups, mean litter size was similar to that for controls.

Sex ratio was unaffected by treatment.

In the 30 mg/kg/day group, there was a higher number of stillborn (male and female) pups and dead (female) pups than in the controls. The difference reached statistical significance in female pups. In the 10 and 3 mg/kg/day groups, the numbers of stillborn and dead pups were similar to that for controls.

There were no malformed pups at birth in any group.

3.2.1.2 Pre-weaning period
Viability (on day 4 postpartum), survival (on days 7 and 14 postpartum) and lactation (on day 21 postpartum) indices were comparable in all groups.

3.2.1.3 Post-weaning, gestation and lactation periods
No deaths occurred during the post-weaning and gestation periods.

One female (No. 1109, 3 mg/kg/day group) was sacrificed for procedural reasons (litter less than six pups) on day 4 postpartum. At necropsy, absence of mammary tissue development was noted.

3.2.2 Clinical signs

No compound-related clinical signs were observed in the F_1 generation.

3.2.3 Body weight

3.2.3.1 Pup data at birth and pre-weaning period
In the 30 mg/kg/day group, mean body weight of male and female pups at birth was lower (−8% and −5%, respectively, when compared with controls) and correlated with lower mean fetal weight observed in the caesarean section group at this dose. Mean body weight of male and female pups was slightly lower on days 7, 14 and 21 postpartum (−5% to −8% compared with respective control values) in the 30 mg/kg/day group. These differences did not reach statistical significance.

In the 10 and 3 mg/kg/day groups, mean body weight of pups at birth and during the pre-weaning period was similar to control values.

3.2.3.2 Post-weaning period
Mean body weight was comparable between control and treated groups.

3.2.3.3 Gestation and lactation periods
Mean body weight was comparable between control and treated groups.

3.2.4 Developmental tests

Physical development
Physical development as assessed by the time of onset and completion of the incisor eruption, eye opening, balano-preputial separation or vaginal opening showed no effect that could be attributed to PP 27567.

Functional development
The results of functional development tests (negative geotaxis, auditory and visual functions) were comparable in all groups.

Behavioral development
The results of behavioral tests (locomotor and exploratory activities, and learning and memory abilities) were comparable in all groups.

3.2.5 Precoital interval, mating and fertility indices and pregnancy rate

Precoital interval, mating and fertility indices and pregnancy rate were comparable in all groups. Therefore, maternal treatment with PP 27567 was considered to have no influence on reproductive performance of the F_1 generation.

3.2.6 Gestation length and observations at parturition

Gestation length and parturition index were comparable in all groups and there were no signs of dystocia in any group. Birth index was significantly lower in the 30 mg/kg/day group (-15% when compared with controls). In the 10 and 3 mg/kg/day groups, birth index was slightly lower when compared with controls (-5% and -9%, respectively). However, as these differences did not reach statistical significance and the values remain within the range of our historical control data, they were not considered to be related to the compound.

3.2.7 Necropsy

3.2.7.1 Day 56 ± 3 postpartum
No compound-related macroscopic findings were observed.

3.2.7.2 Males selected for reproductive performances
No macroscopic findings which could be attributed to the test substance administration were observed.

3.2.7.3 Nonmated and non-pregnant females

No macroscopic findings were noted.

3.2.7.4 Mated females which littered

Maternal observation. No maternal macroscopic findings were noted.

Implantation and post-implantation loss. There was no difference between the groups in the mean number of implantation sites. Mean post-implantation loss was significantly higher in the 30 mg/kg/day group. In the 10 and 3 mg/kg/day groups, mean post-implantation loss was slightly higher when compared with controls. However, these differences did not reach statistical significance and the values remained within the range of our historical control data and, therefore, they were not considered to be related to the compound.

3.3 F_2 Generation

3.3.1 Mortality

There was no effect of treatment of the F_0 animals on the F_2 litter size. In the 30 mg/kg/day group, mean litter size was slightly lower, but this decrease did not reach statistical significance and was considered to be spontaneous.

Sex ratio was unaffected by treatment of the F_0 animals.

There was no dose-related trend in the number of stillborn and dead pups.

One male pup in the 3 mg/kg/day group showed abnormal flexure of hindpaws. This isolated observation was considered an incidental finding and was not attributed to treatment of the F_0 parents.

Survival index on day 4 postpartum was similar in all groups. There was a slight decrease in the survival index on day 7 postpartum for male pups in the 30 mg/kg/day group which was not statistically significant and not considered treatment-related. In the 10 and 3 mg/kg/day groups, survival index on day 7 postpartum was similar to that for controls.

3.3.2 Clinical signs

There were no clinical signs attributable to treatment of the F_0 animals.

3.3.3 Body weight

Mean body weight at birth was similar in all groups. In the 30 mg/kg/day group, mean body weight was slightly lower when compared with controls on days 4 and 7 postpartum (−4% to −9%, respectively). These differences were not considered to be related to PP 27567. In the 10 and 3 mg/kg/day groups, mean body weights on days 4 and 7 postpartum were similar to control values.

3.3.4 Terminal necropsy

No macroscopic findings which could be attributed to the test substance administration were observed.

4 Conclusion

At 30 mg/kg/day, PP 27567 induced adverse parental effects including salivation, lower food intake and body weight gain, slightly lower fertility index and pregnancy rate, and a slight increase in gestation length. These effects were associated with mild effects in the F_1 generation, as indicated by lower mean fetal body weight, delayed fetal ossification, a slight decrease in birth index, and lower pup body weight at birth and during the pre-weaning period.

At 10 mg/kg/day, with the exception of salivation in a few F_0 animals, no adverse effects were observed in the F_0, F_1 or F_2 generations.

At 3 mg/kg/day, no adverse effects were observed in the F_0, F_1 or F_2 generations.

In conclusion, the reproductive and developmental no-effect level of PP 27567 under the conditions of this study is 10 mg/kg/day.

References

Altman J. and Sudarshan K. (1975) Postnatal development of locomotion in the laboratory rat. *Anim. Behav.*, **23**; 896–920.

Butcher R. E., Wootten V. and Vorhees C. V. (1980) Standards in behavioral teratology testing: test variability and sensitivity. *Teratog. Carcinog. Mutag.*, **1**; 49–61.

Dawson A. B. (1926) Note on the staining of the skeleton of cleared specimens with Alizarin Red S. *Stain. Tech.*, **1**; 123–124.

EEC Council Directive (1975) 75/318/EEC, dated May 20, 1975 (O.J. No. L147 of 9.6.75).

EEC Council Directive (1983) 83/570/EEC, dated October 26, 1983 (O.J. No. L332 of 28.11.83).

EEC Council directive (1986) 86/609/EEC, dated November 24, 1986 (O.J. No. L358 of 18.12.86).

Gad S. C. and Weil C. S. (1989) Statistics for Toxicologists, Principles and Methods of Toxicology, 2nd edition, 1989, A. Wallace Hayes, Raven Press, 435–462.

Report PP 674 (1993) Teratology study of PP 27567 in the rat by the oral route with plasma level determination. Poisonous Prose, Inc.

Report PP 684 (1993) Teratology study of PP 27567 in the rabbit by the oral route with plasma level determination. Poisonous Prose, Inc.

Report PP 711 (1993) 6-Month oral toxicity study in rats. Poisonous Prose, Inc.

Ryan P. C., Whelan C. A. and Fitzpatrick J. M. (1988) The vas deferens count: a new accurate method for experimental measurement of testicular exocrine function. *Eur. Urol.*, **14**; 156–159.

Salewski E. (1964). Färbemethode zum makroskopischen Nachweis von Implantationsstellen am Uterus der Ratte. *Arch. Exp. Path. Pharmakol.*, **247**; 367.

US Federal Guidelines (1985) Laboratory Animal Welfare Act (1966) (PL 89-544) as amended in 1970 (PL 91-579), 1976 (PL 94-279) and 1985 (PL 99-198).

Vorhees C. V., Butcher R. E., Brunner R. L. and Sobotka T. J. (1979) A developmental test battery for neurobehavioral toxicity in rats: a preliminary analysis using monosodium glutamate calcium carrageenan, and hydroxyurea. *Toxicol. Appl. Pharmacol.*, **50**; 267–282.

Weil C. S. (1970) Selection of the valid number of sampling units and a consideration of their combination in toxicological studies involving reproduction, teratogenesis or carcinogenesis. *Fd. Cosmet. Toxicol.*, **8**; 177–182.

Zbinden G. (1981) Experimental methods in behavioral teratology. *Arch. Toxicol.*, **48**; 69–88.

APPENDIX 1: Materials and Methods

A1.1 Test and Control Articles

The bulk compound, identified as PP 27567, batch CA 9128000, had a purity of 100%.

The titer of the test article was considered to be 91.6% as free base. The doses referred to throughout this report are expressed in terms of PP 27567 as free base.

The test article was administered as an aqueous suspension containing 0.5% methylcellulose and 0.1% polysorbate 80. Three concentrations for oral dosing were prepared daily or weekly and were administered at a dosing volume of 2 ml/kg/day to achieve dose levels of 3, 10 or 30 mg/kg/day. The vehicle for the test article and control article was water containing 0.5% methylcellulose and 0.1% polysorbate 80. The control article was administered at a dosing volume of 2 ml/kg/day.

The homogeneity and stability of the formulations were satisfactory for the range of concentrations used in this study. Samples of formulations were taken during the study and analyzed for achieved concentrations. The results were close to nominal concentrations and never exceeded a 10% variation.

A1.2 Test System

Male and female Sprague-Dawley rats of the Crl:CDr(SD)BR strain approximately 7 weeks (males) and 9 weeks (females) old at the beginning of treatment were used in this study. The animals were COBS (Cesarean Originated Barrier Sustained) and VAF (Virus Antibody Free). The rat was selected because it is a recognized animal model for this type of safety evaluation study. The Charles River CD strain of rat was used because of the background data available on this strain in our laboratory.

Animals were sequentially delivered, examined physically prior to acceptance in the study, and allowed one week acclimatization. They were then randomly allocated to a dose group where they were individually identified.

A1.3 Housing and Care of Animals

The animals used in this study were handled and maintained in accordance with the requirements of the EEC Guideline (1986) and US Federal Guidelines (1985). Compliance with the above legislation was ensured by adhering to the standards set forth in the Guide for the Care and Use of Laboratory Animals, DHHS Publication No. (NIH) 86-23, revised 1985.

Animals were housed in environmentally controlled rooms and assigned to individual stainless-steel cages in order to minimize possible inter-group differences due to environmental factors. Animals were housed in stainless-steel wire cages throughout the F_0 pre-pairing, the pairing period and from day 35 postpartum to the end of the pairing period for the F_1 generation. Females allocated to the postnatal phase were housed in Makrolon-bodied cages with stainless-steel wire lids and sawdust for bedding.

The animals were allowed free access to a commercially available pelleted diet DSC01 (batches 30804, 30917, 31011, 31215, 40120, 40217 and 40414) supplied by Diet Supply Co., and to filtered tap water.

Copies of the relevant certificates of analysis for sawdust, diet and water have been filed in the research center archives.

A1.4 Experimental Design

The design of this study was consistent with EEC Council Directives (1975 and 1983).

Two hundred and eighty-eight animals (144 males and 144 females) were randomly divided into 4 groups of 36 males and 36 females.

Only F_0 rats were treated: males for 28 days pre-pairing, throughout pairing and up to necropsy, and females for 14 days pre-pairing and throughout pairing, gestation and lactation.

Observations included mortality, clinical examination, food consumption, body weight and macroscopic examination at necropsy.

Twenty F_0 females per group were euthanatized on day 20 of gestation for examination of their uterine contents, including external, visceral and skeletal examination of fetuses. The remaining females were allowed to litter and rear their young to weaning on day 21 postpartum. The physical and functional development and behavior of the F_1 generation were evaluated on standardized litters. On day 58 ± 2 postpartum, 1 male and 1 female per litter were selected for subsequent evaluation of reproductive performance following pairing and the observation of the F_2 generation up to day 7 postpartum.

A1.5 In-life Observations

A1.5.1 Mortality

All animals were checked daily.

All animals found dead or those euthanatized prior to scheduled euthanasia were subjected to a thorough macroscopic examination of the visceral organs to identify the cause of death or morbidity. For females the number of implantation sites in the uterine horns was also recorded.

A1.5.2 Clinical examination

All animals were examined daily.

A1.5.3 Body weight

Males were weighed weekly. Females were weighed weekly until mating and then on days 1, 3, 6, 9, 12, 15, 18 and 20 of gestation and on days 1, 4, 7, 14 and 21 postpartum for those allocated to the parturition phase. Pups were weighed on days 1, 4, 7, 14 and 21 postpartum and weekly thereafter.

A1.5.4 Food consumption

Food consumption was determined weekly for males and females (F_0 generation) during the pre-pairing period and twice weekly for F_0 females from day 1 of gestation to day 13 postpartum. Daily food consumption was calculated for each interval.

A1.5.5 Assessment of reproductive performance (F_0)

After the pre-pairing period, each female was placed with a male for a maximum of 21 consecutive days. Vaginal smears were carried out daily during the pairing period up to mating for all females in order to establish estrus cycle and mating. The day a copulation plug (in the vagina or under the cage) and/or spermatozoa in the vaginal smear was detected was designated day 0 of gestation. The time between initial pairing and detection of mating (precoital interval) was recorded.

If mating was not detected during this period, females were maintained for approximately 2 weeks, at the end of which they were euthanatized. Uterus and ovaries were sampled for histological examination and the presence of implantation was checked by the Salewski staining method (Salewski, 1964).

At the end of the pairing period, sperm collection was performed (vas deferens method) after anesthesia in 10 males/group having mated. Sperm count, motility and vitality parameters were recorded (Ryan *et al.*, 1988).

A1.5.6 Lactation examination (F_0)

During the parturition period, females were observed at least twice daily. Gestation length was recorded as well as any signs of dystocia.

A1.5.6.1 Litter size
The number and sex of live, dead, stillborn and malformed pups were recorded at birth. Stillborn and dead pups were identified using a lung flotation test.

A1.5.6.2 Culling
Culling within sex was performed on day 4 postpartum to obtain 8 pups per litter (4 males and 4 females, where possible). Litters containing less than 6 pups were discarded.

A second cull was performed after the last post-weaning test (on day 58 ± 2 postpartum) to obtain 2 pups per litter (1 male and 1 female, where possible), and a minimum of 15 males and 15 females per group for assessment of reproductive performance.

A1.5.6.3 Examinations on day 4 postpartum (F_0)
F_1 pups were examined and the following recorded for each litter:

- number of live and dead pups
- individual sexes
- examination of individual pups

A1.5.7 Developmental tests

The timing of pup development was assessed on a total litter basis by recording the days on which the onset and completion of the parameter occurred or the performance on a defined day (Altman and Sudershan, 1975; Vorhees *et al.*, 1979; Butcher *et al.*, 1980; Zbinden, 1981).

Physical

- Incisor eruption: eruption of the upper incisor(s) through the gum from day 7 postpartum
- Eye opening: separation of the upper and lower eyelids from day 11 postpartum
- Balano-preputial separation: from day 40 postpartum
- Vaginal opening: separation of the vaginal edges from day 30 postpartum.

Functional

- Negative geotaxis: assessment of a pup's ability to turn and face uphill on an inclined plane (15°) within 30 seconds from day 4 postpartum
- Auditory function (startle reflex): assessment of a pup's ability to respond to a sudden sharp noise from day 10 postpartum
- Visual function (pupillary reflex): assessed by examination of pupil closure in response to a bright source of light on day 19 postpartum.

Behavioral

A water-filled M maze was used to evaluate learning ability on day 42 ± 3 postpartum and memory 7 days later under the same conditions (1 male and 1 female per litter). The time taken by each pup to swim through the maze in six successive trials was measured. A maximum of 60 seconds was allowed for each trial, and pups were considered to have failed if they exceeded the time limit. Improvement in swimming time was taken as an indication of learning ability.

Locomotor and exploratory activities were evaluated on day 49 ± 3 postpartum (1 male and 1 female per litter) during a 9-minute test using a Columbus Optovarimex 3. Output data included distance traveled, resting time, ambulatory time, stereotypic time and number of rearings.

A1.5.8 Development and reproductive performance (F_1)

Following completion of the final behavioral test, F_1 rats were selected from each group for assessment of their reproductive performance. Rats were at least 10 weeks old when pairing took place (see subsection A1.5.5), and sibling pairings were avoided.

During the parturition period, females were observed at least twice daily. Gestation length was recorded as well as any signs of dystocia.

A1.5.8.1 Litter size

The number and sex of live, dead, stillborn and malformed pups were recorded at birth. Stillborn and dead pups were identified using a lung flotation test.

A1.5.8.2   Culling
Culling within sex was performed on day 4 postpartum to obtain 8 pups per litter (4 males and 4 females, where possible). Litters containing less than 6 pups were discarded.

A1.5.8.3   Examinations on day 4 postpartum
Pups were examined and the following recorded for each litter:

- number of live and dead pups
- individual sexes
- examination of individual pups.

A1.6   Terminal Examinations

A1.6.1   Necropsy

A1.6.1.1 F_0 and F_1 males
After pairing, F_0 males and F_1 males selected for assessment of reproductive performance were euthanatized by CO_2 inhalation and subjected to macroscopic examination.

The testes and epididymides were weighed in pairs. These tissues were collected and fixed for possible microscopic examination.

A1.6.1.2   Non-mated F_0 and F_1 females
Two weeks after the end of pairing, non-mated females were euthanatized. The presence of implantation sites was checked by the Salewski staining method (Salewski, 1964). Uterus and ovaries were collected and fixed for possible microscopic examination.

A1.6.1.3 F_0 females of caesarean section phase (F_0)
Rats were euthanatized on day 20 of gestation by CO_2 inhalation and were subjected to macroscopic examination. Their uteri and ovaries were removed and the following parameters were recorded:

- number of corpora lutea in each ovary
- number and distribution of implantation sites
- number and position of early and late uterine deaths
- number and distribution of viable fetuses in each uterine horn.

Uteri from apparently non-pregnant females or individual uterine horns without visible implantations were checked for evidence of implantation sites using the Salewski staining technique (Salewski, 1964). Uterus and ovaries were collected and fixed from non-pregnant females for possible microscopic examination.

External examination of fetuses. The following parameters were recorded:

- weight and sex of viable fetuses
- external abnormalities of viable fetuses, their placentae and fetal envelopes.

Individual viable fetuses weighing less than 2 g were classified as 'small fetuses'. Each viable fetus was euthanatized by a subcutaneous injection between the shoulder blades of about 0.1 ml sodium pentobarbitone solution and examined in detail by dissection. All viable fetuses were identified individually using numbered tags.

Internal and skeletal examination of fetuses. Approximately half of the fetuses were examined by dissection immediately after necropsy. The head and heart, where possible, were fixed in Bouin's solution for examination by serial sectioning and dissection. Following evisceration, the skeletons of the remaining fetuses were examined after staining using a modified Dawson technique (Dawson, 1926).

A1.6.1.4 F_0 and F_1 females allowed to litter

Following weaning or total litter death, the females were euthanatized by CO_2 inhalation and subjected to macroscopic examination. The number of implantation sites was recorded.

Any female failing to produce a litter on day 25 postcoitum was euthanatized by CO_2 inhalation and subjected to macroscopic examination for the presence of implantation sites. Uterus and ovaries were collected and fixed from non-pregnant females for possible microscopic examination.

A1.6.1.5 F_1 pups

After the second cull, non-selected young were euthanatized by CO_2 inhalation and subjected to macroscopic examination.

A1.6.1.6 F_2 pups

F_2 pups were euthanatized on day 8 ± 1 postpartum and subjected to macroscopic examination.

A1.6.2 Microscopic examination

No microscopic examination was performed as no macroscopic changes were observed.

A1.7 Calculations

Calculations (Weil, 1970) were performed using a SAS (Statistical Analysis System) software package. Group mean values were calculated for each recorded parameter.

Mating performance and fertility

For each sex and group the following were calculated:

Male mating index =
$$\frac{\text{Number of males having inseminated at least 1 female}}{\text{Number of males paired}} \times 100$$

Female mating index =

$$\frac{\text{Number of mated females}}{\text{Number of paired females}} \times 100$$

Male fertility index =

$$\frac{\text{Number of males having produced at least 1 pregnant female}}{\text{Number of males having inseminated at least 1 female}} \times 100$$

Female fertility index =

$$\frac{\text{Number of females with evidence of pregnancy}}{\text{Number of mated females}} \times 100$$

A1.7.1 Caesarean data

Group mean values with standard deviations were calculated for each litter and each group.

Group mean values for the size of litters, uterine deaths, early and late resorptions were calculated using either of the following means:

- Mean 1: All pregnant females surviving to term bearing evidence of implantation (including total litter resorptions).
- Mean 2: All pregnant females surviving to term bearing viable fetuses.

Mean 2 has more significance when group size is small as the data would be influenced by the presence of a single total litter resorption. Mean 1 is more accurate when several females exhibit total litter resorption. For mean litter and fetal weights and the number of fetal observations, only Mean 2 was calculated.

Pre-implantation loss (Number of corpora lutea − Number of implantations) was calculated for each female. When the number of implantations exceeded the number of observed corpora lutea, pre-implantation loss was taken as 0. Pre-implantation loss includes losses due to non-fertilization of ova and early post-implantation deaths (i.e. those occurring up to days 8–9 of gestation).

Post-implantation loss (Number of implantations − Number of viable fetuses) was calculated for each female. Post-implantation loss covers only the period between days 8–9 and 20 of gestation and does not include the first 2–3 days post-implantation, as any death occurring in this phase would leave no visible remains on day 20.

Group mean implantation loss values were calculated as means of individual values.

Group fetal observation values (external, internal and skeletal) were expressed as a percentage and calculated from the formula:

$$\frac{\text{Number of fetuses with a particular observation}}{\text{Number of pregnant females in the group}} \times 100$$

A1.7.2 Postnatal data

Post-implantation loss (Number of implantations – Total number of dead or live pups at birth) was calculated for each female. Post-implantation loss covers only the period between days 8–9 and the end of gestation and does not include the first 2–3 days post-implantation, as any death occurring in this phase would leave no remains visible on day 21 postpartum.

Group mean implantation loss was calculated as a mean of individual values.

Live birth index was calculated as follows:

Live birth index =

$$\frac{\text{Number of live pups at birth}}{\text{Number of implantations}}$$

Postnatal indices were calculated as follows:

Viability index =

$$\frac{\text{Number of live pups on day 4 postpartum}}{\text{Number of live pups on day 1 postpartum}} \times 100$$

Survival index on days 7 or 14 =

$$\frac{\text{Number of live pups on day 7 or 14 postpartum}}{\text{Number of live pups on day 4 postpartum}} \times 100$$

Lactation index on day 21 =

$$\frac{\text{Number of live pups on day 21 postpartum}}{\text{Number of live pups on day 4 postpartum}} \times 100$$

The postnatal indices were calculated for each litter and then per group for these values. The calculation of the number of living pups on day 4 postpartum was established after culling, except for the viability index.

A1.8 Statistical Methods

Statistical analysis (Gad and Weil, 1989) was performed on the individual values for dam parameters and by sex on the mean values for the litter and pup data.

Differences between the treated and control groups were tested using a decision tree to select an appropriate hypothesis-testing procedure.

Parametric data, i.e. food consumption, body weight, body weight change, absolute and relative organ weight, gestation length, litter size, fetal weight, number of implantation sites, pre- and post-implantation loss, physical and functional development and behavioral tests were analyzed in the following way. A Bartlett's test was carried out in order to verify the homogeneity of variance, and then:

- when the variances were found to be homogeneous, an overall Analysis of Variance was carried out by means of the F test followed, when significant, by multiple and pairwise comparison of the group means using the Dunnett's test;

- when the variances were found not to be homogeneous, the overall comparison of the groups was carried out using the Kruskal–Wallis test followed, when significant, by multiple and pairwise comparison of the group means using the Wilcoxon Rank Sum test.

The final toxicologic interpretation of data considered other factors such as dose–response relationships, biological plausibility and consistency.

Categorical data, i.e. mating and fertility indices, pregnancy rate, parturition and live birth indices, percentages of stillborn or malformed fetuses, mortality of pups, postnatal indices, pupillary reflex test and the water maze test were analyzed by means of the Fisher's Exact test.

A1.9   *Archives*

All raw data, specimens and other study documents pertaining to this study will be stored in the respective research center archives.

Using References

The following are our recommendations for using references in toxicology reports.

12.1 Journals

12.1.1 References in the Text

Mention the authors and the year of publication: "(Dawson and Dupont, 1972)". Cite first author + *et al.*" for three or more authors: "(Dawson *et al.*, 1985)". If there are 2 or more references, list them by alphabetic order of the authors and then by increasing year, e.g. "(Dawson *et al.*, 1926; Dawson *et al.*, 1929; Lindsay, 1971)".

12.1.2 References in the References Section

List the authors and year of publication, title, journal, volume number, first-page–last-page, by alphabetic order of the authors and then by increasing year.

Example: Dawson A. B., Dupont C. D. and Durand E. F. (1985) Note on the staining of the skeleton of cleared specimens with Alizarin red *Stain. Tech.*, 1; 123–124.

For two or more references of the same author and same year, list them as follows: "Dupont (1994a)" and "Dupont (1994b)".

12.2 Books

12.2.1 References in the Text

State the author and the year of publication: "(Keenan, 1958)". For two authors, refer to both: "(Hannah and Blow, 1987)". Cite the principal author + "*et al.*" for three or more authors "(Blackwell *et al.*, 1952)".

12.2.2 *References in the References Section*

List the author and year of publication, title of the part of the book, "In:" Editor's surname, "ed.",. title of the book, edition number (2nd or above), place of publication, name of publisher, volume number, chapter number or page numbers if specific pages are cited.

Example: Kavet J. (1976) Trends in the utilization of influenza vaccine: an examination of the implementation of public policy in the United States. In: Selby P, ed. *Influenza: Virus, Vaccines, and Strategy*, 2nd ed, Orlando, Fla.: Academic Press Inc.; 297–308.

12.3 Unpublished/In-house Reports

12.3.1 *References in the Text*

Give the report number and the year of signature: "(Report PP 93-221, 1993)".

12.3.2 *References in the References Section*

Cite the report number, the year of signature, the title and the name and location of the testing facility.

Reports PP XX-XXX are listed by increasing report year and/or report number.

Example: Report PP 93-016 (1993) PP 27567: Two-week oral toxicity study in rats. Drug Safety Laboratories, Poisonous Prose Inc., Littlebrook, Surrey, UK.

13

References and Recommended Reading

ALLEY, M. (1987) *The Craft of Scientific Writing* (Englewood Cliffs, N.J.: Prentice-Hall International).

AMERICAN NATIONAL STANDARDS INSTITUTE, INC. (1979a) *American national standards for the preparation of scientific papers for written or oral presentation*. ANSI Z39.16-1979 (New York: American National Standards Institute, Inc.).

(1979b) American national standards for writing abstracts. ANSI Z39.14-1979 (New York: American National Standards Institute, Inc.).

ANONYMOUS (1982) *The Chicago Manual of Style*, 13th edition (Chicago: The University of Chicago Press).

(1990) *Mosby's Dictionary, Medical, Nursing and Allied Health*, 3rd edition (St. Louis, Mo.: Mosby).

BLACK, H. E. (1994) Design and writing of the preclinical safety report, *Toxicologic Pathology* 22 (2), 202–5.

COMMITTEE OF GRADUATE TRAINING IN SCIENTIFIC WRITING (1989) *Scientific Writing for Graduate Students* (Bethesda, Md.: Council of Biology Editors, Inc.).

COUNCIL OF BIOLOGY EDITORS STYLE MANUAL COMMITTEE (1983) *CBE Style Manual. A Guide for Authors, Editors and Publishers in the Biological Sciences*, 5th edition (Chicago, Ill.: Council of Biology Editors, Inc.).

DAY, R. A. (1991) *How to Write and Publish a Scientific Paper*, 3rd edition (Cambridge: Cambridge University Press).

DEVLIN, J. (1987) *A Dictionary of Synonyms and Antonyms* (New York: Warner Books).

FARR, A. D. (1985) *Science Writing for Beginners* (Oxford: Blackwell Scientific Publications).

FOWLER, H. W. (1968) *A Dictionary of Modern English Usage*, 2nd edition (rev. by Sir Ernest Gowers) (Oxford: Oxford University Press).

GOPEN, G. D. and SWAN, J. A. (1987) The science of scientific writing, *American Scientist*, 78, 550–8.

GOWERS, E. (1986) *The Complete Plain Words* (revised edition by S. Greenbaum and J. Whitcut), 3rd edition (London: HMSO).

GREGORY, M. W. (1992) The infectiousness of pompous prose, *Nature* 360, 11–12.

HODGSON, E., MAILMAN, R. B. and CHAMBERS, J. E. (1988). *Macmillan Dictionary of Toxicology* (London: Macmillan).

MATTHEWS, B. R., LEE, R. M., EISEN, S. M. and DEWS, I. M. (1994) *How to Write an*

Expert Report, B. R. Matthews (ed.) (MCRC Group, Romford, Essex RM7 7DA, UK: Rostrum Publications).

SCIENTIFIC ILLUSTRATION COMMITTEE, COUNCIL OF BIOLOGY EDITORS (1988) *Illustrating Science: Standards for Publication* (Bethesda, Md.: Council of Biology Editors, Inc.).

SHERMAN, T. A. and JOHNSON, S. S. (1992) *Modern Technical Writing*, 5th edition (Englewood Cliffs, N.J.: Prentice Hall).

ZBINDEN, G. (1987). *Predictive Values of Animal Studies in Toxicology Testing*, CMR Annual Lecture 1987 (Carshalton, Surrey, UK: Centre for Medicines Research).

Index